D1882325

INFANT MORTALITY AND MATERNAL MORTALITY (SOCIO-ECONOMIC CAUSES AND DETERMINANTS)

INFANT MORTALITY AND MATERNAL MORTALITY
(Socio-Economic Causes and Determinants)

PADMA SETH

GYAN

Infant Mortality and Maternal Mortality Socio-economic Causes and Determinants

Published with Permission obtained from the Planning Commission

Rs. 750

© Padma Seth

ISBN: 978-81-212-1021-8

All rights reserved. No Part of this book may be reproduced in any manner without written permission.

Published in 2009 in India by
Gyan Publishing House,
23, Main Ansari Road, Darya Ganj,
New Delhi-110002
Phones : 23282060, 23261060
Fax : 011-23285914
E-mail: books@gyanbooks.com
Website: www.gyanbooks.com

Lasser Type Setting by: Quick Media, Delhi
Printed at : Young Art Press, Delhi - 92

Dedicated to My Mentor

Dr. Smt. Durgabai Deshmukh

CONTENTS

1

INTRODUCTION

The Planning Commission vide its letter No. 15012/07/06-SER dated 6th September 2006, has entrusted the Indian Trust for Innovation and Social Change a Research Project entitled, 'Infant Mortality and Maternal Mortality Socio-Economic Causes and Determinants.'

This Research Study is based on empirical inputs provided by this Trust's investigators and its allied Research institutions located in different States. This study covers a number of districts of the States of Tamil Nadu, Andhra Pradesh, Maharashtra, Rajasthan, Uttarakhand and Haryana.

This study also involves personal interviews and discussions with several MLAs, MPs, Women Leaders, Social Welfare Boards, prominent members of NGOs etc. I was privileged to have detailed conversations with some former and current Cabinet Ministers of the Union Government and some learned Judges and Public figures of the States surveyed in this study.

The Broad Methodology

(*a*) Field investigations, empirical surveys, direct interviews with villagers specially women, young mothers, traditional dais, Anganwadi workers, the Auxiliary nurse midwives, doctors and Self Help Groups, Panchayat Sarpanchas and members.

(*b*) Extensive scanning of published material on the subject.

(*c*) Scanning of a few previous and current Five Year Plan Provisions to reduce IMR and MMR. A special attention was given to the Mid-term reviews not only of the Planning Commission but also of Reports of some Ministries viz. Ministry of Health and Family Welfare, Ministry of Women and Child of the Centre and the States; National Rural Health Mission, important local feedback from Panchayat Raj reviews and a few members of the Panchayats of the concerned States.

(*d*) This project also drew the benefits of scanning international literature on this subject in other Asian and African countries.

(*e*) Internal Researchers attached to us continuously focussed their attention in internal brainstorming sessions, to seek answer to a "MAJOR QUESTION" What *new* can we do to supplement the existing Schemes and Programmes on reducing and reversing wherever possible, the existing picture of mortality.

Secondly, is it not IMR/MMR, interalia, because of the lack of empowerment of women in India, can we either through new direct methods or a number of indirect strategic approaches, to invigorate connected and unconnected systems as well as many sub-systems; as also other behavioural determinants, practices superstition and decadent traditions; so that the strategic synergy could converge to a single goal of decelerating IMR and MMR. All this is reflected in the subsequent Report under five key facets as given below :

(*i*) Aspects of Infant Mortality (IMR)

(*ii*) Aspects of Maternal Mortality (MMR)

(*iii*) Some prominent features of socio-demographic environmental factors.

(*iv*) Key Constraints : Social-economic-cultural-environmental-administrative, nutritional, health delivery services.

(*v*) Aspects of empowerment of women and the girl child to have a say on important matters of their lives and survival.

Behind all our deliberations, questionings, discussions and formulation of new direct or indirect inputs for the search of alternate policy supplements, we have tried to remind ourselves constantly of the key sociological features pertaining to India. These are as follows :

(*a*) India is a large human system.

(*b*) Poverty status of India prevails all over the country.

(*c*) Indian society exists simultaneously in different centuries with its concomitant living patterns and practices. (there are still people in our country, some of whom are in the 2nd century India, 9th century and some others are knocking at the emerging 21 century India).

(*d*) Arising from the above three factors, we display a unique cultural pluralism wherein superstitions co-exist with science.

(*e*) We are also practising technological plurality. India similarly lives in bullock cart economy as well as space era. (Here hardly any technology vanishes or is replaced totally by technological advancements. We are a museum piece of technological non-violence).

To conclude, in order to grasp the merit of the report, as a prefatory observation, one has to say the following: (1) A great deal of remedial measures to curb IMR/MMR as the Indian society exists today, will be those which are already known and are being implemented through the various policy provisions, official grants-in-aid and through the modern inputs, as and where they have reached.

We will be re-emphasising even earlier schemes and ideas, which are not new, and which are well known. There is nothing profound about this except that they are still useful and relevant in places and therefore, deserve to be continued.

Nevertheless, all our efforts of social reform through education, legislation, higher literacy rates, better personal income and general overall development in the health and governance mechanisms, still remain inadequate to demolish taboos, practices and traditions which constitute an ugly spot on 21 century modern India.

We need not comment on the enforcement failures be it that of a local administration, the Police system or the,"law enforcement" mechanism, to crack down on such elements of society who pretend as keepers of decadent social norms and practices. In passing, can we just add that even judiciary could have helped and has not quite lived up to the expectations of those who suffer caste, community, religious and other unfortunate traditional adverse practices involving horrific murders as INFANT MORTALITY and MATERNAL MORTALITY.

Finally, this report provides a qualitative and quantitative input. We have tried to stay away from the statistical jugglary and by no stretch of imagination pretend to provide magical recipes to liberate a large nation like ours from IMR/MMR. Our advice, in remedial policy options, cannot constitute "the last word on the subject".

I thank every one, too numerous to be named here for their technical and intellectual contribution. I particularly thank Dr. Syeda Hameed, Member, Planning Commission and the Advisors of the Planning Commision, for giving this Trust an opportunity to carry out this study.

In any case, the problem of IMR & MMR is part of the Indian, "Social Complexity". To totally bring it down we need to take vigorous direct and indirect systemic reform steps.

No research survey, including this, can hardly put forward the definitive steps on this subject, realizing that we are seeking a, "mind-set", change for a billion plus people.

In any case, it is high time, we took not one but several, "first steps" some of them have been recommended here as we have to walk a thousand miles to bring down IMR/MMR in India.

(PADMA SETH)
Executive Director ITISC and
Director of this Project
Former Member National Commission of Women
& Senior Consultant, UNICEF.

2

INFANT MORTALITY

Aspects of Infant Mortality : A Social Malaise

In the context of Infant Mortality, the study of Six States of Andhra Pradesh, Tamil Nadu, Maharashtra, Rajasthan, Uttarakhand and Haryana, we have focussed on the qualitative research-survey. It was indeed laborious and time consuming. From the information and data collected it revealed that the root cause for stagnating and perpetuating of infant mortality has been, the rural belief system, their cultural practices, and many a superstitions and taboos. These in short, influenced their rural health behaviour and health choices. This complex mixture of myth and magic even today continues to cast its spell on the rural people. The casualties are children and women. For a thorough examination of the village psyche and its populace. Socio-economic, cultural and demographic features, it is necessary to understand the root causes accelerating Infant Mortality.

Infant mortality is an indicator of the health status not only of infants, but also of the whole population and of their poverty ridden social and economic status in the country. They face excessive vulnerability, as underprivileged, to a hostile environment and suffer, malnutrition and serious health problems; All this leads to high rates of infant mortality and morbidity. *Infant mortality i.e. deaths under one year of age in a year per 1000 live births, is an important indicator of child health and development.*

A decade and a half ago, it was recorded that there was rapid decline in infant mortality, but it has apparently stagnated for the past five to six years. The current period

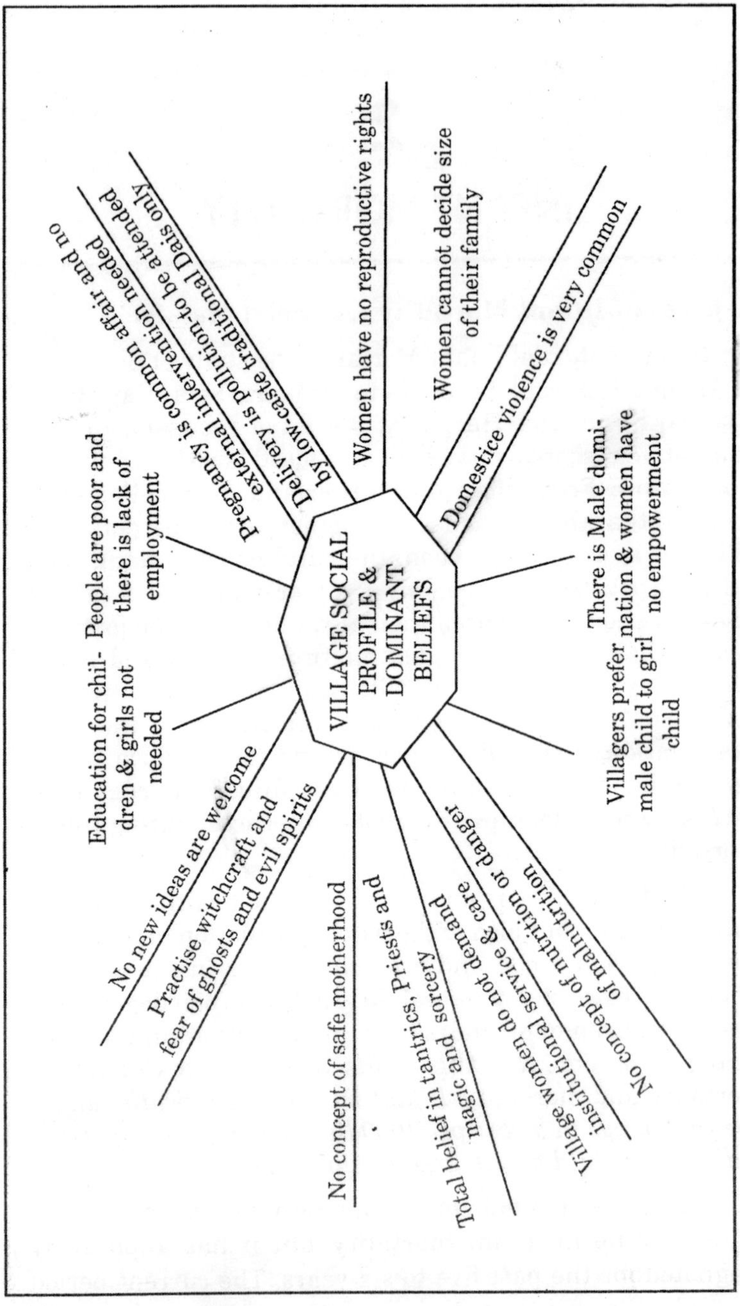
VILLAGE SOCIAL PROFILE & DOMINANT BELIEFS
Women have no reproductive rights
Women cannot decide size of their family
Domestice violence is very common
There is Male domination & women have no empowerment
Villagers prefer male child to girl child
No concept of nutrition or danger of malnutrition
Village women do not demand & care institutional service or danger
Total belief in tantrics, Priests and magic and sorcery
No concept of safe motherhood
Practise witchcraft and fear of ghosts and evil spirits
No new ideas are welcome
Education for children & girls not needed
People are poor and there is lack of employment
Pregnancy is common affair and no external intervention needed
Delivery is pollution-to be attended by low-caste traditional Dais only

of slow decline has made it difficult to achieve the National Child Mortality goals by 2000.

The reduction in infant and child mortality was declared as the major goal of our official strategy to achieve Health for All by 2000. One of the main objectives of the Government of India's Population Policy 2000 was to reduce the present level of high infant mortality and bring it down to less than 30 per 1000 live births by the year 2010. As per the figures available in 2002, Infant Mortality rate has been 63 per 1000, which is reported to have come down to 59 in 2005-6. However, Neonatal Mortality declines rapidly from about 70 in 1981 to 40 in 2001. This was attributed to the focus given by the planners and policy makers to a reduction stance of Neonatal Mortality.

Social Profile

A pertinent question however, we need to ask is: "why is the decline in Infant mortality rates slowing"? Many research studies conducted so far have explored the causes and determinants of infant Mortality in India. The key findings, besides pointing at the medico-clinical causes, indicate that the Socio-Economic factors like household income, female education, access to health services and immunization programmes are important determinants to assess status of infant mortality. Some studies also identify a strong inter-relationship between mortality, fertility and gender bias. Others, emphasise, how demographic factors impact on infant mortality, and vaguely touch on many other socio-economic factors that have contributed to high infant mortality. These include proximate factors, such as medical care of the mother during antenatal period, care at birth, preventive and curative care in the post natal period. Maternal factors, i.e. age at marriage, age at first birth, parity and birth intervals, household and community level factors: They felt that better water, drainage, sanitation, housing could increase access to a minimum package of essential services and could significantly reduce infant mortality rates. Besides, reproductive health services, perinatal care, improved breast-feeding practices, immunization, home based treatment of diarrhoea were also suggested.

An elaboration of the social profile of the villages is necessary to explain how socio-economic factors are the main causes and determinants behind IMR. *Community norms, values and practices are assiduously followed by the rural folk. Their perception of various developmental indicators and their views on women, pregnancy, child birth etc. are given below:*

1. Modern education is thought to be redundant and hence not pursued.
2. There is total absence of scientific temper; also non-acceptance of new ideas is the norm.
3. Pregnancy and child birth are considered a natural phenomena that require no medical intervention or attention.
4. Girls are to be consigned to home based chores and they need to adhere to the imposed patriarchical norms and customs.
5. Women are not supposed to make decisions on any issue in the family.
6. People have boy preference as against girls; because they believe that boys will alone can atone their earthly faults and become an "old age" aid.
8. Girls do not deserve attention since they have to go away to her husband's family. (They are called, a *Paraya Dhan* (others property and wealth).
9. Deliveries are considered as pollution and hence low-caste dais alone are thought fit to handle the deliveries.
10. There is no concept of safe-motherhood practices.

11. Total belief in Tantrics, faith healers, Ojha's and priests.
12. Tardy or no co-operation offered by villagers to governmental health and educational programmes. This credibility gap still fails to disappear but continues.
13. Majority of people suffer from poverty and lack of employment as there are no sustainable vocations, available for villagers locally.
14. There is no concept of nutrition among the villagers nor do they understand the dangers of malnutrition.
15. Crude ways of handling the new born and no understanding by Dais on dangers of infection persists.
16. Absence of toilet facilities, sanitation and hygiene, particularly menstrual hygiene is totally absent.
17. Belief in witchcraft, sorcery and magic abounds in the nooks and corner of India.
18. No concept of clean drinking water exists. Non-availability of potable drinking water universally in the country.

Economic Causes and Determinants : Behind Infant Mortality

(i) Economic factors influence infant mortality in a big way. Child survival depends on the ability of the parents to offer good care. If they are in the BPL category, their capacity for child care is minimal. Also, illiteracy and ignorance of the needs of child care are glaring. Many studies have highlighted that the degree and quality of survival of the infant lie with the quality of care providers. The numerous economic factors have both direct and indirect impact on the survival of children and on infant mortality. Some of them are as follows :

(a) The status of economic development of the household/village.

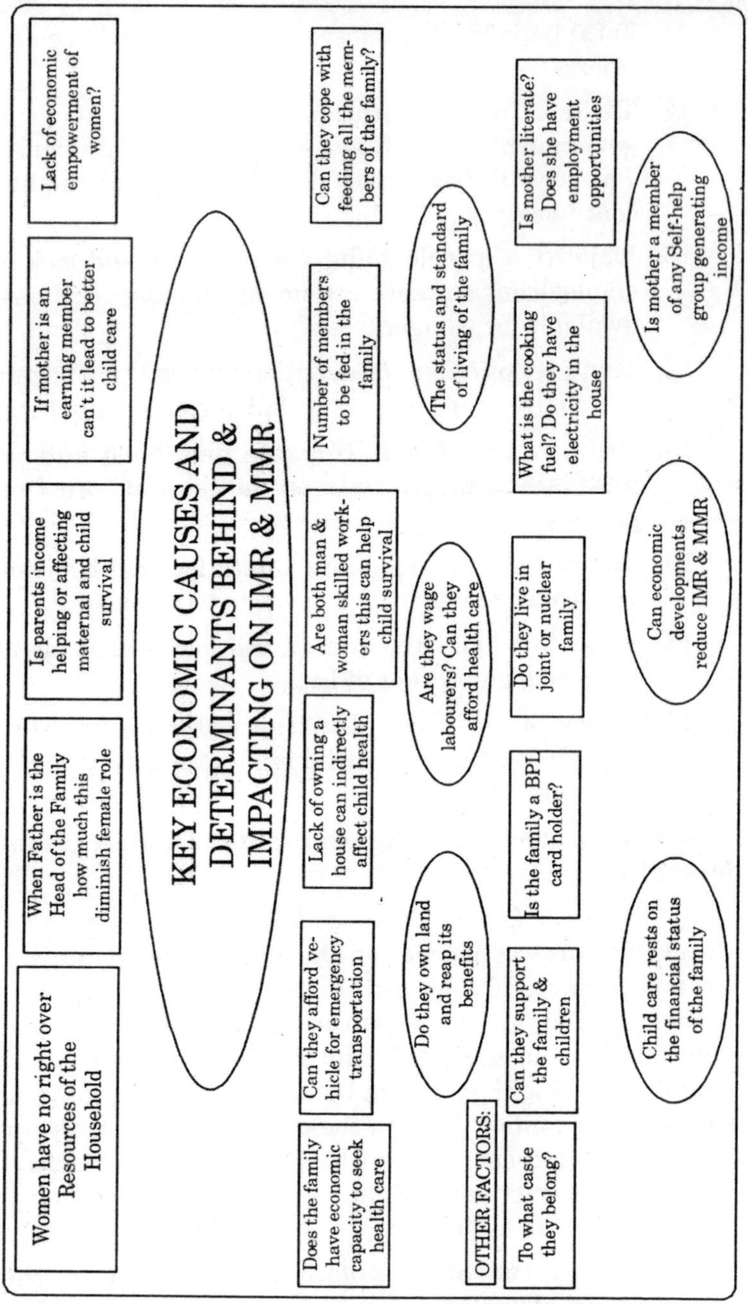
KEY ECONOMIC CAUSES AND DETERMINANTS BEHIND & IMPACTING ON IMR & MMR
Women have no right over Resources of the Household
When Father is the Head of the Family how much this diminish female role
Is parents income helping or affecting maternal and child survival
If mother is an earning member can't it lead to better child care
Lack of economic empowerment of women?
Does the family have economic capacity to seek health care
Can they afford vehicle for emergency transportation
Lack of owning a house can indirectly affect child health
Are both man & woman skilled workers this can help child survival
Number of members to be fed in the family
Can they cope with feeding all the members of the family?
Do they own land and reap its benefits
Are they wage labourers? Can they afford health care
The status and standard of living of the family
OTHER FACTORS:
To what caste they belong?
Can they support the family & children
Is the family a BPL card holder?
Do they live in joint or nuclear family
What is the cooking fuel? Do they have electricity in the house
Is mother literate? Does she have employment opportunities
Child care rests on the financial status of the family
Can economic developments reduce IMR & MMR
Is mother a member of any Self-help group generating income

(b) Poverty and its various deleterious manifestations.

(c) Number of families holding a BPL (below poverty line) card.

(d) Number of members to be fed in the family.

(e) Is father the head of the household?

(f) Household income. Occupation of the parent.

(g) Is the mother an earning member?

(h) Type of house they live in? Own house or is it on rent?

(i) Is the father a cultivator or a labourer?

(j) Standard of living of the family.

(k) Does the family has any vehicle for transportation?

(l) Are both man and woman skilled workers?

(m) To which caste do they belong?

(n) Dependant or self-supporting?

(o) Nuclear family or joint family.

(p) Social participation in economic activity.

(q) Land holding/farm power.

(r) Is the mother educated.

(s) Financial ability to seek medical care.

(t) Is the mother, member of any self-help-group?

(u) Women's access to earning and employment opportunities.

(v) Any specific coping strategy used to ensure food security, health and nutrition to the whole family?

(w) The type of cooking fuel used by the family.

(x) Do they have electricity in the house?

(y) How helpless and dependent the women are, on the mercy of the family and their assistance.

The general standard of living and lifestyle of people, the persisting poverty in every household, the feeble capacity of the head of the household to provide food for all the members and women and girl children of the family, and allied environmental and social factors do influence adversely the infant mortality in a community. Factors which are remote to the existing life styles, e.g., the availability and utilization of medical health facilities, also fall under socio-economic imperatives.

The education of the mother is considered important for the health outcome of children. The empirical evidence and health statistics do show that the educated mothers are usually healthier and give birth to healthier babies. They also provide healthier environment to children and their own health care. Even the illiterate but informed women can take better care of the child. Majority of them do not have "Akshar Gyan". Accessing official health services do involve financial expenditure. Earning mother can ensure better investment on infant and child care. Economic factors too are thus important indicators to assess and understand the cause and determinants of infant mortality.

The word economic is too heavy a word to depict the assorted darkness that, people living a penniless and a marginal existence. Their existential status cannot be captured by Plan panel's economic indices. The Planning Commission's Technical notes may highlight a macro-setting but it cannot totally capture the misery of millions of men and women of our village and tribal settlements, who have neither a social persona or an economic persona or even an awareness persona, of what is good and what is bad in terms of child health. Not only that, their only life guiding thrust comes from what they have heard, from their forefathers or what they have seen them practising. It is an unfortunate and tragic gap and chasm in appreciation of this stark naked truth which diminish the values of the well informed modern programmes and recipes of welfare and

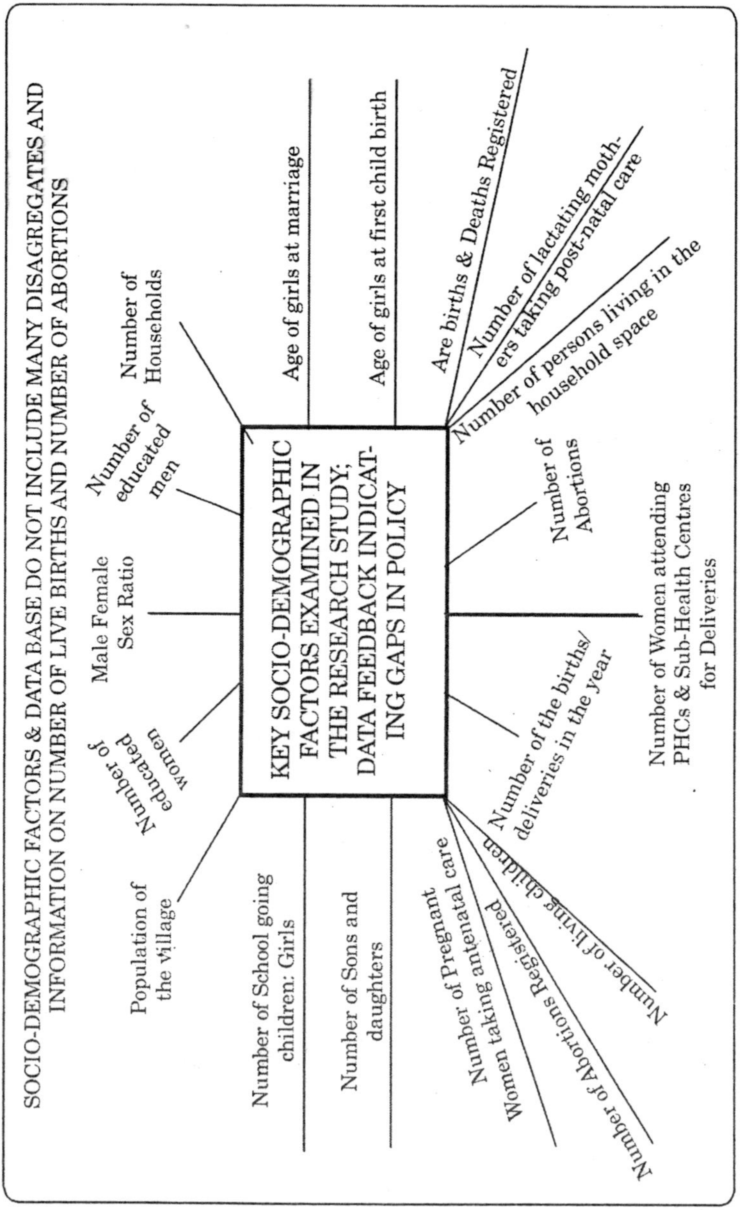
SOCIO-DEMOGRAPHIC FACTORS & DATA BASE DO NOT INCLUDE MANY DISAGREGATES AND INFORMATION ON NUMBER OF LIVE BIRTHS AND NUMBER OF ABORTIONS
KEY SOCIO-DEMOGRAPHIC FACTORS EXAMINED IN THE RESEARCH STUDY; DATA FEEDBACK INDICATING GAPS IN POLICY
Population of the village
Number of educated women
Male Female Sex Ratio
Number of educated men
Number of Households
Number of School going children: Girls
Age of girls at marriage
Number of Sons and daughters
Age of girls at first child birth
Number of Pregnant Women taking antenatal care
Number of Abortions Registered
Number of living children
Number of the births/ deliveries in the year
Number of Women attending PHCs & Sub-Health Centres for Deliveries
Number of Abortions
Number of persons living in the household space
Number of lactating mothers taking post-natal care
Are births & Deaths Registered

causes and determinants lie more in the village practices and belief systems and taboos. We need to extend and step-up modern medicines, for cures to ailments but it is extremely important to also tackle the attitudes and behaviour of the people steeped in superstition and fear of modern medicine and medicare. The root cause of non-acceptance is because of lack of familiarity, lack of awareness and fear of the unknown on the part of villages and tribals and remote area denizens.

Can we say that our current medical indices and social indicators have been fully taken into account, the above mentioned features of poverty and superstition that guides the life of rural and of tribal area inhabitants.

Socio-demographic Factors (Also called Maternal Factors)

Demographic factors also fall under the over all socio-economic ambit. For purposes of enumeration and for reasons of measurement, quantification and classification, they are brought under what is called, "demographic factors". The following demographic factors are the outcome of the socio-economic causes.

There is difference between indicative change and absolute accomplishment. Statistics do not cover it. It may be a mere indicator of an ameliorative change, but does not represent the total local practices. The following factors least recorded amply bear the above statements :-

1. Age at marriage - Marriage of adolescent girls below 18.
2. Age of woman at conception.
3. Maternal age at birth - when mother is not mature.
4. Live birth or foetal death.
5. Preceding birth interval.
6. Number of persons living in one room.
7. Number of previous abortions.

8. Number of living children/sons.
9. Ante-natal care if attended by ANMs or Dais.
10. Non-registration of births, marriages and deaths.
11. Adoption of family planning practices by men and women.
12. Place of delivery.

For the items cited under the above demographic factors; these too become intense due to rural beliefs and cultural practices. The practice of giving away children and adolescents girls in marriage before the legal age of marriage at 18, has lead to early conception, that is common knowledge. The low birth weight babies are the outcome. Both congenital deformities and underdevelopment of the child are some of the handicaps that the young and immature mother has to handle. There is no data available on the number of adolescent marriages solemnized since there is no law on compulsory registration of marriages. However, infant mortality, both neonatal and post neonatal are common occurrences because of early marriages followed by early motherhood. How can we ensure safe motherhood and child care in such a situation? Added to these this lack of data on crucial maternal factors inhibits authentic assessment of the unmeasurable propensity of risk to the infant survival and mortality.

As shown by various empirical research studies, the proper childcare processes cannot be overlooked in order to save infants from mortality, until and unless we can ensure safe motherhood and child care. In such circumstances, the unscientific and faulty infant feeding practices and depriving the young mother of nutritious food after delivery, are sad and unfortunate manifestations of local cultural practices. A birth interval, which means a spacing between the first child and the following ones is an important factor not only for mother's health but also in deciding the prospects of child survival. Frequent deliveries by the anaemic mothers leads to continuous malnutrition and infant mortality. Also deprivation due to food intake based on households and community beliefs and practices do threaten both the maternal and the child survival.

For medical termination of pregnancy (MTP) though legally permitted and to be conducted by specified medical practitioners, but a majority of pregnant women seek help only of dais and quacks in the village. In a majority of such cases crude ways used for abortions do result in maternal mortality and killing of the foetus. Abortion though indicated as a demographic factor is often not recorded. *Hence any record maintained of infant mortality, without record of abortions give inadequate and a distorted picture.* At present oral pills are available for easier abortions. **It is regretted that qualitative research like the present study is handicapped for want of sufficient official data on miscarriages and abortions, besides foeticide and infanticide.**

It is not a practice in our villages that the pregnant women of the villages go in for antenatal care thrice before delivery. Post natal care is a misnomer altogether. Most of the deliveries that take place are at home and they do not utilize the antenatal and post natal facilities or receive required sanitary health care from the local midwives.

Most women and families prefer to have a male child and not a girl child. This boy preference does reveal the discriminatory story of the girl child which persists for her through out her life cycle from her birth, growth', adolescence, marriage and motherhood etc. All family and social norms are duly obeyed by women. The demographic indicators are part and parcel of the village culture and practices that have contributed to infant mortality.

Environmental Factors

The public health depends a great deal on environmental factors. The number of studies conducted by both the Indian scholars and the foreign researchers do touch on

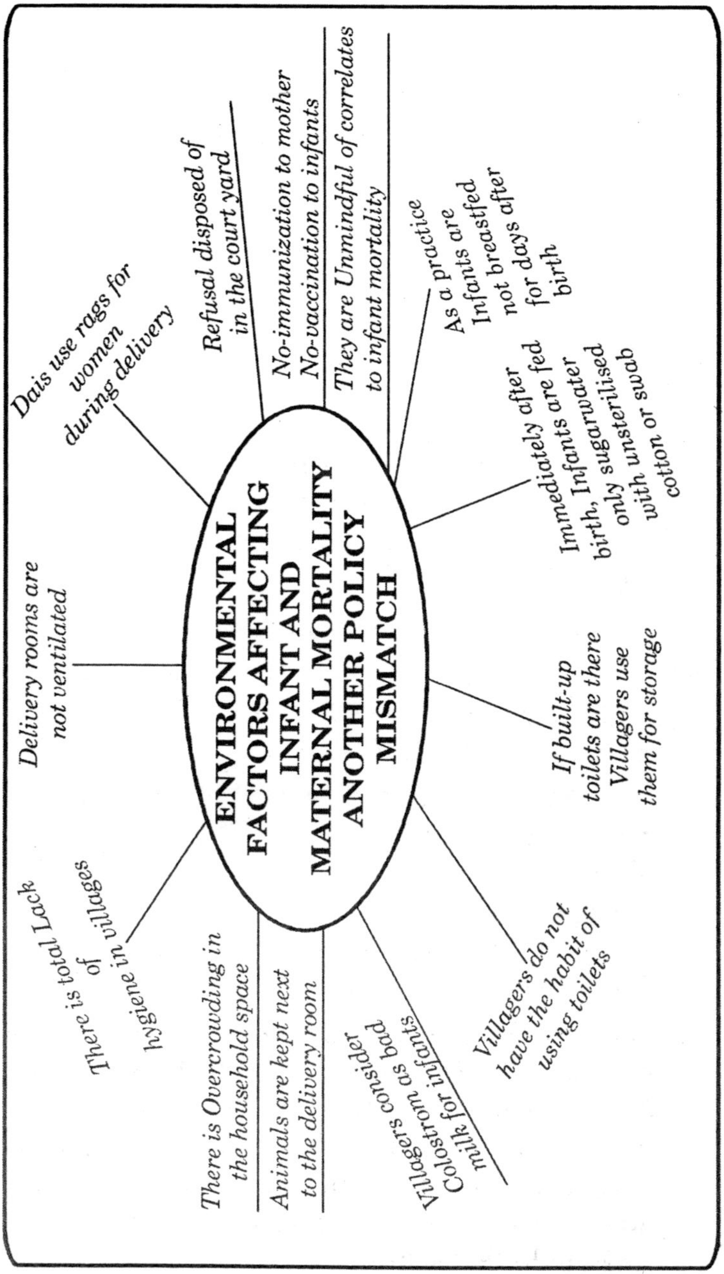
ENVIRONMENTAL FACTORS AFFECTING INFANT AND MATERNAL MORTALITY ANOTHER POLICY MISMATCH
There is Overcrowding in the household space
Animals are kept next to the delivery room
There is total Lack of hygiene in villages
Delivery rooms are not ventilated
Dais use rags for women during delivery
Refusal disposed of in the court yard
No-immunization to mother
No-vaccination to infants
They are Unmindful of correlates to infant mortality
As a practice Infants are not breastfed for days after birth
Immediately after birth, Infants are fed only sugarwater with unsterilised cotton or swab
If built-up toilets are there Villagers use them for storage
Villagers do not have the habit of using toilets
Villagers consider Colostrom as bad milk for infants

environmental sanitation; but more as a corrollary to the medical factors and as supplementary cause for infant mortality. The lack of hygiene and sanitation are taken as part of village life. Local initiatives are mostly absent in cleaning up their habitat. All blame is put on government for the unsanitary conditions of one's own village. Our team's local interrogations revealed local belief in the God given life wherein the environmental conditions, such as, access to safe water and sanitation facilities, access to electricity and use of clean cooking fuel were not deemed as part of their Karma. This lack of rationality and local insensitivity has important health impact on young children. Above all it is a failure of the State apparatus that could not provide these basic amenities even after sixty years of independence. Some of the familiar factors, catalogued by us were :

1. Overcrowding and lack of ventilation, sanitation and hygiene.
2. Rampant spread of infectious diseases.
3. Lack of care during and after child birth and the traditional habit of giving "Gutti" to infant reveals no child care after birth.
4. Near total indifference to hygiene for the infant. The delivery room where the child was born was totally plugged of all holes to protect the male child from 'evil eye'.
5. Family planning measures adopted were conditional to the survival of children.
6. Ignoring of immunization and vaccination. Many pregnant women confessed that their mothers-in-law do not allow them for these procedures.
7. Waste disposal in their own courtyard results in infection. This reflects the total absence of public health authorities and their unconcern for environmental health.

8. Lack of drainage in the village lanes. This shows absence of political will for necessary action.
9. Villagers do not use toilets - but they go to the fields. This only shows how they refuse to change their habits.
10. Use of dirty rags during delivery. This is highly dangerous, but the idea that delivery is pollution as per villagers belief is the main reason for such practices.
11. Feeding sugar water to the infant with unsterilised swab. This is doubly harmful (i) by depriving the child of mothers milk and (ii) refusing nutrition that will enhance immunity to the child.
12. Animals kept adjacent to the delivery area.

A prerequisite for living in a healthy habitat is good ventilation, sanitation and personal hygiene. How is it possible in a room that has to accommodate all the members of the household and some times even the cattle? Do these purely fall under medical issues? Are'nt they not part of village lifestyles and also their economic necessity. It is both ignorance of the need for sanitary conditions and the lack of resources to provide ideal shelter for the pregnant and lactating mother. Some researches on religious practices and ethnicity also reinforce the above facts as causes and determinants behind infant and maternal mortality.

Lack of Potable Water Supply is a Key Public Health Issue

The lack of adequate water supply is an urgent issue. But there is no one to monitor the supply of water or usage or wastage of available water. There exists competition amongst villagers to draw as much water as possible by each household unmindful of the requirements of other villagers. A sense of belonging to ones village and one community too is an issue that needs attention. Caste discrimination as to who will draw water first from which well or taps, stares at us as an evil discriminatory practice that lingers on even today. Civic consciousness being absent, no one removes the puddles of water in front of their homes that harbours mosquitoes, spreads malaria and other infections. Such behaviour may not be attributed to cultural practice but to the ignorant and indifferent people and their way of life. *Well-being of others does not seem to be a community value: Villagers rich or poor are solely concerned with their own interest and well being.*

Role of Self Help Groups

Improvement in human ecology shows a ray of hope by women voluntarily forming themselves into Self Help Groups. These groups not merely focus on their economic betterment but act as an almoner in times of emergency. For example, when a woman in labour with complications and has to be rushed to a medical centre or to a hospital, Women from these self-help groups deposed before us that they pool money for bearing transportation charges for helping women in distress. In village Harsaroo in Gurgaon district of Haryana, the village SHG has offered help to pregnant women by taking them to the government hospital or private clinics; thus they assisted in saving the unborn from mortality and also helped the woman from maternal mortality. At the instance of District Rural Development Agency (DRDA) SHGs are getting formed. And they become eligible for getting sizeable amount as loan to start economic enterprises. In Madurai and Salem districts of Tamil Nadu SHG's have pooled money and have received four times the loan from the Bank. They have sponsored education of poor girls with the loan money. This is one way to stop women from infanticide of girl child causing IMR.

Under the rural development project (DRDA) (Swarna Jayanti Gram Swa Rozgar Yojana) women are encouraged to form themselves into groups of 15 or more where in they contribute a monthly sum ranging e.g. of Rs. 50/- or more.

Once the group is able to collect a sizeable amount of, e.g., Rs. 5000 they are entitled to get six times loan from the bank on easy pay back instalments and on easy interest. These SHGs then start one or more economic and income earning activities and then distribute the profits amongst the members; at times in emergencies they do lend an amount sought by one of the members who is needy. *These self help groups have brought change in the village help-line.* A small dent is being made by the formation of Self Help Groups of women whose members act as social workers and volunteers at times of emergency. They should be multiplied in all States; they will act as a resource and arrange transport for the pregnant woman, mother or infant to be rushed to the hospital, or to the health centres or to private doctors in the neighbourhood. Our researchers met the SHGs in villages Harsaroo in Haryana and in Magudanchavadi in Salem district of Tamil Nadu and felt inspired by local SHG's activities.

ALL VISIBLE CONSTRAINTS IN REDUCTION OF IMR

Role of National Rural Health Mission

The National Rural Health Mission of 2005 with the Reproductive Child Health II programme promises better infant and maternal health and reduction in infant mortality, than the earlier safe motherhood programme under RCH-I. The existing infrastructure of Primary Health Centres and the Sub-centres with the introduction of ASHA worker is a welcome innovation. But to make a new entrant's life and work in the village successful, special efforts have to be made to bring under one umbrella, all the different agencies functioning in the village i.e. ICDS project with its Anganwadis, the Primary Health Centres and the Sub-centres, their medical practitioners, nurses and ANMs and ASHA have to work cohesively and in collaboration with one another. The ideal situation will be to work under the leadership of an enlightened village Panchayat. Once linkages are established, the work environment will improve and interaction will become effective. Each functionary will have to know ones individual and collective responsibilities. The constant presence of these functionaries working by rotation and harmoniously in the village will enhance better local participation in our efforts to reduce IMR. Such a collective effort is the true answer for human development that can ensure better survival of infants and reduce infant mortality.

The many expectations as cited above in reality are absent even today. ASHAs have yet to be appointed in many health centres. Though they are to be trained by doctors in the civil hospital, their actual role and performance is very limited. They are neither trained in nursing nor are they professionals. They can at best act as conduits between the pregnant women and the institutional machinery, i.e. the Primary health centres and the sub-centres. Some times they do rush the women in emergency to the Community Health Centres or hospitals also, even though they are situated at a distance. ASHA's effective and timely performance can contribute to the reduction in IMR.

Caste/religion/class/poverty: The complex village culture has an added dimension by way of caste, religion and class on one side and poverty and deprivation on the other. There is lack of employment avenues leading to poor households suffering economic disabilities. Coordination amongst the various service providers in the village have to be brought in, to improve the condition of families and thus help in improving the health status of infants/children, pregnant and lactating mothers.

The Infrastructure and Glaring Gaps

The ICDS structure with the Anganwadi workers is expected to serve as a forum in the village where creche for infants and preschool and nutrition is to be provided for children of three to six years age. Here the pregnant and lactating mothers are also to be attended to for their antenatal and postnatal care. Adolescents come to receive nutritious snacks, folic acid and iron tablets. In southern states of Tamil Nadu and Andhra Pradesh, midday meals are given to children, pregnant and lactating mothers who come to the Anganwadis. This is a great incentive for children and mothers who are below poverty line families to visit the Anganwadis. In northern Indian states, dry *nashta* is given. Our team of field staff and I personally saw those white maize balls which are hard to bite. Even this poor and so-called nashta is still attracting children with their mothers. This can be the first step and an opportunity for local functionaries to interact with women of the village and counsel them on the best health practices and child care. The primary health centres and sub-centres are expected to work in close collaboration with Anganwadis. But the work area of ANMs is dispersed and they have to make periodic visits to centres and to the villages around. Their main job is to immunize and vaccinate pregnant mothers and children and to offer help in deliveries, emergencies and antenatal care. But the ANMs visit a village sub-centre only on a fixed day in a month. The occasional visits by the health centre staff and not to find them in the village daily, creates apprehension in the minds of the villagers. Therefore they revert back to their old practice of depending on the traditional methods provided by the local faith healers.

In such a scenario there are no medical staff nor doctors available to the villagers at times of need. This discourages the rural folk in accessing medicare services. In Umrale gaon in Nashik district of Maharashtra, our team and I personally went to the PHC and met the patients admitted for not only delivery but even those who had tubectomy also. Such centres are far and few in numbers. Trudging long distances, mud roads prove to be a disincentive for villagers seeking better health care.

The conceptual framework of the health delivery services in the villages is a welcome first step. But many gaps remain in the recruitment policies of the Anganwadis, the ANMS, the doctors and the multipurpose workers. The Anganwadi worker - a tenth pass girl/woman from the very village where she will work first gets recruited. But she hardly has proper training. With this handicap, she is supposed to attend to many chores i.e. keeping a number of Registers. There is no *creche* for 0-3 year age group. Secondly, the ANGW is also expected to visit women's homes, and meet the pregnant women and enquire about the infants health and counsel them on a variety of subjects in particular, food and nutrition intake and the iron folic acid tablets to be taken regularly. Due to lack of proper and adequate training, the Anganwadi worker finds her work exhausting and unmanageable.

Another handicap in the village is the caste segregation. In Hayatpur village in district Gurgaon of Haryana State the Sarpanch an SC refused to interact with an anganwadi worker, a non SC. It is for the local governance to take leadership role and monitor the working of the various functionaries in health, i.e., the ANMs, schools and public health sector. But if these public functionaries do not see eye to eye with each other, the National Rural Health Mission cannot function satisfactorily to arrest the rise in IMR/ MMR. What is required is *'change'* in the recruitment and training policies of the Anganwadi workers, the ANMs and ASHAs. The Panchas and Sarpanchas too need orientation and training. Besides, all these village level workers and functionaries, need "on the job training" continuously, for one and a half to two months, without any break.

In many of these PHCs we found ANMs appointed on contractual basis. The ANMs though are expected to stay in the village and be able to attend to women and infants but they often live in distant villages and, therefore, are not able to attend to emergencies. Villagers are left to their own fate thus.

The NRHM scheme is lofty but the implementation machinery, if we can call it as a synthesized entity, has many holes and gaps. The Panchayatiraj personnel, including the elected ones, is almost a challenge. Many Presidents of the Panchayats who have become neorich by selling away their prime cultivable lands do not show interest in attending to any training programme. They do not attach any value to learning or training. Only money making/earning is considered important and worthy of their attention.

To sum up, unless administrative requirements of fine tuning of recruitment policies and rules are taken up with a sense of urgency, the laudable objectives of the NRHM will be in peril. Both in Maharashtra villages and in Andhra Pradesh as also in Uttarakhand, Rajasthan there were no ASHAs yet recruited. In Haryana, we could see a very few ones are in place; some of the Dais also offered to act as ASHAs.

States do not seem to follow the guidelines of the Centre as they are free to frame their policies and rules. Their bureaucratic machinery can no more deliver goods at the ground level. *What is imperative is to have a multi-sectoral approach that is needed to be adopted and a central monitoring mechanism is essential to make the Mission's goals attainable. With this limping infrastructure available in the villages and with the indifferent Panchayat raj functioning, unaware of their role and responsibilities, and the ill-equipped and ill-staffed Primary Health Centres and sub-centres do not send healthy signals.* In such circumstances, the villagers withdraw themselves and find refuge in their own dilapidated, archaic, socio-economic determinants that cannot salvage IMR and MMR.

Habits and attitudes do not change overnight by erecting health and educational infrastructure at the village level by starting the Primary Health Centre/Sub-centre and a primary school cannot automatically change the die hard habits, behaviour and attitudes of the village community. Definitely, an educated mother will be able to understand the prerequisites for child-care and if she is also an earning member she can contribute, to better growth of the child.

Lack of Concern and Indifference of Villagers

In most villages it was observed that a great many individual homes are swept clean. But all the waste water is thrown out in the street/lane. The roads are thus flooded. There is no drainage system in the village. Village health environment adversely influences infant and child mortality. Even the Sarpanch and Panches have shown little, if any concern to approach the public health authorities to get their villages in shape.

The Statement that Development is not a surety for infant survival is very true. Haryana is a rich state where industrial development has touched heights. But the public health system has taken a back seat. A technical issue like drainage can easily be solved if there is political commitment and a will to engage experts to fix the drainage. Mo-bikes and latest cars zoom in the narrow lanes of the villages; but the level of education of people and their civic consciousness is abysmally low and is almost nil. Women's status remain poor and static. Even school educated girls once they are married, are not allowed the freedom of movement or decision making even in women's personal matters.

To Sum Up

Based on our limited study, we do feel emboldened to seek an answer from the planning and health policy of the government whether the following life expectancy indicators of infants/children have been checked, monitored and achieved?

They are:

- The age of the girl at marriage
- The age at first child birth
- Delivery conducted at home/ or at the PHC/Hospital
- Fertility status of the woman
- Spacing of birth of the children
- Acceptance of family planning devices by the couple
- Woman's education/and level
- Woman's employment and economic status
- Woman's reproductive and child health rights.
- Woman's empowerment.

However, whatever be the new remedial measures we may introduce in the 11th and 12th Five Year Plans, let us also pay attention to the dangers to infant survival and find ways and means to cope with to alter or totally eliminate them:

- Irrational rural beliefs and village health culture.
- Villager's lack of faith in modern medication.
- Rural faith and belief in external i.e. supernatural factors, the evil spirits and evil eye.
- Cultural practices affecting the birth of the girl child, her retarded growth, foeticide.
- Infanticide and villager's preference for sons as against girl child.
- Dowry demands, child marriages and adolescent - pregnancies.

- Blind sacrifices of children based on predictions by the priests.
- Low value attached to women whether it is for their productive work or their reproductive obligations.
- Unhealthy environment, lack of sanitation/potable water and stinking drainage.
- Lack of awareness of nutrition, dangers of malnutrition. (known but not fully catered to.)
- Caste and religious discriminations and crude practices, deserve new legislative remedy, besides the fine tuning and effective management practices which are region specific.
- Unfair customary practices depriving the pregnant, lactating mother and infants of nutrition and food.

3

MATERNAL MORTALITY

Maternal mortality is an issue of great concern both in the national and international health agenda. For many decades, there had been a single focus 'on fertility regulation' it viewed women's health with a narrow perspective, as limited to their reproductive system between 15-45 years of age. Mothers health in the past Indian Policy has been particularly of measures to improve infant and child health we are happy that now the current health policy lays additional emphasis on reducing maternal mortality.

What is Maternal Mortality

The maternal mortality has been defined by WHO as death of a woman while pregnant or within 42 days of termination of pregnancy, irrespective of the cause of death (and) is intended for countries that wish to identify deaths occurring in pregnancy, child birth upto 6 weeks after the end of pregnancy but where the cause of death cannot be identified precisely. (WHO cited in Royston, Mauldin, 1994).

How do we Assess the Status of Maternal Mortality?

The tragedy of maternal mortality affects mainly the poorer sections of society. In our research study conducted in the villages of Gurgaon and Rewari districts in Haryana we were informed that it is the chowkidar of the village who keeps the record of births and deaths in the village. We do feel astonished that important records of infant mortality and maternal mortality are kept by a junior village functionary like a chowkidar, who is either illiterate or at best neoliterate. Fortunately, we could find records kept by the Anganwadi worker and ANM of the primary health centres in the villages: i.e. Akera and Kapadivas in Block Daru Heda in Rewari district of Haryana state. They have kept records of pregnant and lactating mothers and also a register showing births and deaths occurred during the year and a year earlier. We could see and examine those available records; so far the registration of births and deaths has not been made compulsory. Hence, the data available from these records on maternal mortality and infant mortality are quite inadequate. The reasons entered in the records for deaths were sketchy, vague and incomplete. This scenario is almost the same in most of the villages we surveyed. It is not at all a habit for villagers to go on their own to the Anganwadis and Primary or Sub-health centres to inform them of births and deaths. Our experience in the State of Rajasthan and Uttarakhand had been worse. In the tribal villages i.e. Rasegaon and Umrale in Maharashtra state (in Nashik district, Dindori taluqa) where the Gram Sewak keeps the record of births and deaths. Here too we found that the Anganwadi worker/ANM make entries in the register and also feed this information from time to time to the Gram Sewak. Again we could see the limitations in keeping of these records.

Women and Health

To understand the causes of MMR and IMR we have to look into the traditional belief about health and disease that villagers in Haryana attribute to the supernatural forces and to the wrath of evil spirits. These ideas were told to our field investigators in the other states too. The attitude of villagers towards health and customary behaviour reflect the rural health culture of the women and the village folk. They have been studied by us in great detail and highlighted. Our findings from the empirical study conducted in the 48 villages in the twelve districts of Six States give us a clear picture of women's health and *the Socio-economic causes and determinants that lie behind Maternal Mortality and Infant Mortality.* These do confirm what has been earlier found in the research publications. It is so believed that "the traditional Indian systems of medicine are male oriented and male dominated. They largely ignore the women's diseases. The only traditional medicine available to women was in the hands of dais who dealt mainly with pregnancy and delivery" (Jeffery et al. 1983). It needs no two opinions to state that what was true in 1983, is due to local customs and tradition is still prevalent in the nook and corners of India. We found this as true in Bassi and Bateri villages of Jaipur district in Rajasthan. Irrespective of the medical system, the prime gap remains in the lack of enough number of maternal delivery shelters.

It may be of some interest to recall here that in the year 1994 when I was a member of the first National Commission for Women, we arranged a programme to celebrate the International Women's Day on the 8th of March at the India International Centre, New Delhi. The then Deputy Director General, Health Services Dr. Raja Ram publicly stated that even if near all the telephone booths are mobilised as a maternal delivery shelters, even then they will be inadequate to cope with the need spectrum of maternal health at the time of deliveries and post-delivery care of mother and child and their safety.

Health Policies : How far Effective?

It may be argued that the above may be yesterday's phenomena; let us turn to today where in India we believe firmly that the Health is a basic Human Right. Besides the Constitution of India provides for equal rights and equal opportunities in all areas to its citizens irrespective of sex, race, caste or religion. Based on these basic tenets, it may be recalled here that the National Health Policy of 1982 was formulated. It came with its overall goal of, "universal provision of comprehensive primary health care services". The shortcomings of the past were traced as, rapid population growth, high mortality among women, infants and children, extensive malnutrition, onset of various infectious diseases and lack of access to rural people of potable drinking water and basic sanitation; the only relief available to women was the untrained traditional birth attendants; earlier the right emphasis on the prevention of maternal mortality was lacking. The poor health situation was looked at by many as the outcome of few and far between the hospital based curative approach to provide health services.

National Campaign on Health for all by 2000

To fulfill the promises made, a national campaign on, 'Halth for all' by 2000 (initiated by WHO) was announced. Instead of building awareness and self-reliance amongst people, this approach by India also some how did weaken the community's capacity to cope with its own health needs. The situation is gradually changing. In three villages by name Thottappanayakanur, Uthappanayakanur and Alligundam of Madurai district in Tamil Nadu today, there are 18 Self Help Groups formed by women to help themselves and other women in need. Under the Tamil Nadu government's Magalir Dittam Scheme, Rs. 10,000 loan was given to individuals to start any enterprise that would earn them a reasonable income to feel independent and take care of their health and that of their children; also to save themselves from maternal mortality. They were also encouraged to access and avail of institutional facilities for deliveries. The village women spoke confidently and said that they feel happy to be economically independent of their husbands and that with their earnings they can take full care of their households. They also take independent decisions to go for sterilization and tubectomy. They also force their friends and other women, to get sterilized after the birth of two children.

But as a contrast we have found that in some of the north Indian States women still feel dependent and are not able to have access to the various government schemes started for the benefit of women and girl children. The above mentioned experience that we had in Madurai villages has been quoted here to show how the economic empowerment strategy has emboldened women to shun archaic values of dependency on the male head of the household. They need not continue to be waiting to receive doles or alms. These Madurai region women have asserted themselves to attend to their reproductive health needs and contribute to the reduction of maternal mortality and infant mortality. But surely we can't say it for women even of Tamil Nadu. Such success stories, however small, need to be replicated State by State.

The Official Assessment of Maternal Mortality

The National Health Policy of 2002, though came with a focus to study and examine the poor health scenario and to face the challenges in the provision of health care in India, the grim picture of maternal mortality persists. Its confirmation came from the Sample Registration Survey of 2003 which brought to notice the high incidence of maternal deaths as 420 per 100.000 live births. This implies that 15% of all deaths among women in reproductive age are pregnancy related. For details see Sample Registration Survey's Maternal Mortality in India 1997-2003, - Trends, causes and risk factors. The Registrar General of India, New Delhi states, "Under the prevailing conditions and the presumption of decline being too linear, the MMR would be around 231 by 2012. Using conservative estimates, the MMR would be 195 by then. Appropriate and strong governmental policies would then be required to meet the targets of NRHM and MDG."

Arrival of the National Rural Health Mission 2005

It is well known fact that many a gap exists between plan targets and its implementation of the same by the governmental machinery.

Our Plan schemes have been very serious on coping with IMR/MMR. The Tenth Five year Plan started with a focus on i.e. social empowerment, economic empowerment and gender justice. This is based on the National Policy on Empowerment of Women (2001). Amongst many monitorable targets adopted for the 10th Five Year Plan and beyond, reduction of Maternal Mortality Rate (MMR) to 2 per 1000 live births by 2007 and to 1 per 1000 by 2012 is significant.

Realising the slow pace of reduction of both Infant Mortality and Maternal Mortality, the National Rural Health Mission was launched by Hon'ble Prime Minister in April 2005.

The NRHM sought to reduce Maternal Mortality (MMR) in the country from 407 to 100 per 100,000 live births and the total fertility rate from 3.0 to 2.1 within the 7 year period of the mission. *The significant feature of the Plan of Action for NRHM is to make the public health delivery system fully accessible and accountable to the community. Having launched with a plan outlay of Rs. 6075.17 crore in 2005-6. NRHM received an increased outlay of Rs.7155.97 crore (RE) as plan funds in 2006-7. This has further been increased to Rs. 9801 crore(BE) in 2007-8.*

Besides, one of the major goals of the Government of India's Department of Health and Family Welfare has been to reduce maternal mortality and morbidity.

The focus has now shifted from individualized interventions to improvement of over all maternal health. This is also a major goal in The Millennium Declaration of the United Nations. The MD goals speak directly of the rights and needs of women and children. It seeks to reduce the maternal mortality by three quarters by 2015.

The UNICEF has pledged support to the Government of India and the State governments in accelerating the second phase of the National Reproductive and Child Health Programme—(RCH II) for the period 2004-2007. *The dilemma is that how in spite of the PLAN outlay, commitment, policy framework and investment on reproductive health, the MMR is not showing signs of reduction ?*

Gender Bias and Health Policy Mismatch?

After all, when health policies and programmes though are focused on women, why do they often perpetuate gender stereotypes and fail to consider socio-economic disparities and other differences among women? Clearly, the health specific policies may not fully take into account the lack of empowerment of women as affecting their health.

The policy stances, and provisions however lofty they may be, yet they fall short of meeting with the realities of the Indian villages. In our research study we have found some quaint contradiction. What we have found is that our policies do not negate catering to the needs of a pregnant woman's health care but prove feeble external assistance. This mismatch situation prevails in majority of the villages that we surveyed. In village Harsaroo and Hayatput in district Gurgaon, which are near the capital of the state within 10 to 16 kilometers away, were devoid of any health care provisions. Local life is too difficult here to get potable water; these villagers have to fetch water from outside the village.

Household after household we heard, as how women are dependent on the male head of the family for all, their needs including food, health, finances for the whole survival and that of the children. We have earlier pointed out how in Tamil Nadu, in Madurai and Salem districts, rural women employed either as farm labour or construction labour, have asserted themselves and gained some freedom of action and of movement than their counterparts in the other Indian States. Even in villages of Maharashtra (of Nashik district and Nagpur district) though the women were engaged in income earning vocations, they lacked freedom even to cook what they wanted. They could not even visit their parents, without the permission of their husbands and in-laws. So we find a disabled woman who cannot by her own volition avail of modern healthcare; In our view it is indeed a mismatch. Such limitations, it has been suggested here, do provide a state of mismatch in availing the benefit of the health policies of the government. Thus the infanticide of girl children is still prevalent amongst the tribals in Salem district of Tamil Nadu as also in Rajasthan and Haryana. The governmental programmes have not yet succeeded in eliminating these abominal practices.

Women Health Care Needs a Holistic Approach

The Tenth Plan has certainly specified monitorable targets for certain indicators of social development in Health, Education and Gender Equality. But the targets remain unreachable so far. Again with the specific focus on reducing maternal mortality, the apprehension was gaining ground that the non-reproductive health needs of women during their pregnancy tend to be neglected. In passing, we could say in the context of a holistic view of women's health.

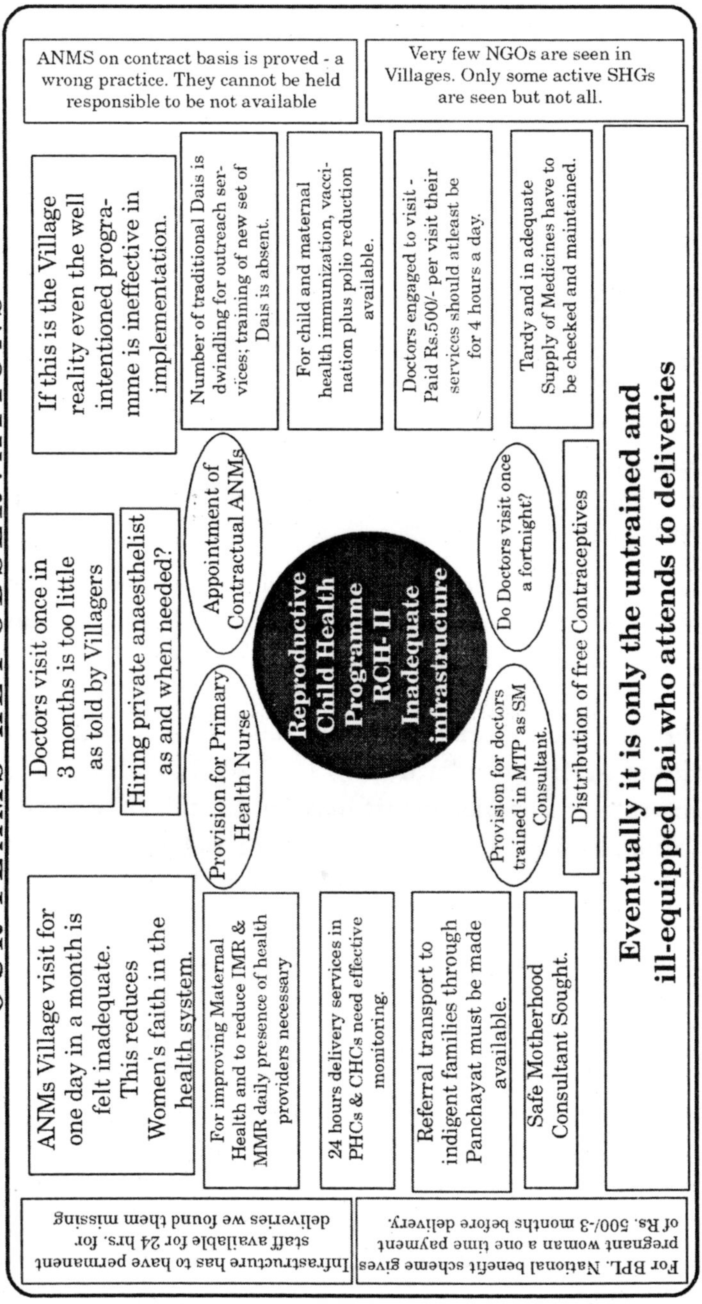
OUR TEAMS KEY OBSERVATIONS
ANMS on contract basis is proved - a wrong practice. They cannot be held responsible to be not available
Very few NGOs are seen in Villages. Only some active SHGs are seen but not all.
If this is the Village reality even the well intentioned programme is ineffective in implementation.
Number of traditional Dais is dwindling for outreach services; training of new set of Dais is absent.
For child and maternal health immunization, vaccination plus polio reduction available.
Doctors engaged to visit - Paid Rs.500/- per visit their services should atleast be for 4 hours a day.
Tardy and in adequate Supply of Medicines have to be checked and maintained.
Doctors visit once in 3 months is too little as told by Villagers
Hiring private anaesthelist as and when needed?
Appointment of Contractual ANMs
Provision for Primary Health Nurse
Reproductive Child Health Programme RCH-II Inadequate infrastructure
Do Doctors visit once a fortnight?
Provision for doctors trained in MTP as SM Consultant.
Distribution of free Contraceptives
ANMs Village visit for one day in a month is felt inadequate. This reduces Women's faith in the health system.
For improving Maternal Health and to reduce IMR & MMR daily presence of health providers necessary
24 hours delivery services in PHCs & CHCs need effective monitoring.
Referral transport to indigent families through Panchayat must be made available.
Safe Motherhood Consultant Sought.
Eventually it is only the untrained and ill-equipped Dai who attends to deliveries
Infrastructure has to have permanent staff available for 24 hrs. for deliveries we found them missing
For BPL. National benefit scheme gives pregnant woman a one time payment of Rs. 500/-3 months before delivery.

It is relevant here also to state the World Bank's view expressed as way back in 1994, that, *"it is useful to consider the entire life cycle when addressing the causes and consequences of women's poor health. This allows for a focus on the particular problems which affect females at different stages of the life cycle and recognizes cumulative effects and life time problems." (World Bank 1994).*

Some Landmark International Views

For instance, the Cairo Conference on Population and Beijing Platform for Action 1995, recognized that women's health involves their emotional, social and physical well being and is determined by the social, political and economic context of their lives, as well as by biology. (UN 1995(1)c).

The WHO estimates suggested that 199000 maternal deaths occurred in South Asia and near 74% were accounted for by India. This amounts to 120000 maternal deaths which is far above the upper range of the Sample Registration Survey for that period (SR 1997-2003). The overall average rate of MMR in India during 1997-2003 has been 24% at this rate of slow decline, it may be difficult to achieve the National Rural Health Mission's target of 100 by 2012 and MDG's 109 as expected by 2015. Thus reduction of maternal mortality is one of the major challenges to improve the overall quality of life. The absence of reliable estimates of MMR makes the process difficult and complex. (SRS-1996) Such a viewpoint is not original a statement. International literature on the subject quotes, "MORTALITY however is not a single factor to be expressed as a single number or index. *The risk of death is something that must be measured in several aspects in many instances.* These measurements might be provided by life tables and if there were enough life tables in existence. (George W.Barclay-Princeton University).

In terms of resource allocation, women's health care has often been channeled through maternal and child health services (MCH). These services are usually limited to aspects of reproductive child health services. They do not cover all other women's health needs. in the past MCH services have been commented upon for putting too much focus on the child. However, motherhood, represents a part of child, women's lives and health needs.

A more holistic approach to women's general and reproductive health needs, may be necessary to create quality of care in health services, to increase womens access to avail of them. What we noticed during our surveys in the villages is that mere allocation *of Funds for health services for villages do not necessarily reach them. This has been a common complaint in all areas of development.* The right mechanism need to be designed and deployed to reach out to the needs of village women and children. Laudable policies seem to remain far away from the intended improvement of physical, social and emotional well being of women.

Socio-Economic Causes and Determinants Prespective behind Maternal Mortality

The issue of maternal mortality can be approached from a number of perspectives, either adopting a health/welfare rationale or a rights based rationale. The Population Conference and the World Conference on Women held in Beijing in 1995 emphasised the importance of women's reproductive and sexual rights as well as the complex, economic, social, political and cultural factors underlying women's health. Thus, looking at maternal mortality in isolation will not yield the right answers.

Let us now turn to our socio-economic research by our field investigators; Whether it is in the villages of

Rangareddy or Chittoor districts in Andhra Pradesh or Jaipur or Jodhpur districts in Rajasthan, Gurgaon or Rewari districts in Haryana, Chamoli or Kumaon of Uttarakhand, Nashik or Nagpur districts in Maharashtra or even Madurai and Salem districts of Tamil Nadu, *the health of Indian women is seen as a chain of a number of linked and gender related concerns that manifest themselves in the socio-cultural, economic, demographic, nutritional, educational, environmental, political, legal and other factors in the traditional Indian society.* Specially younger adolescents are married young and dominated by the in-laws and husband. Their physical movement is restricted. They have no control over their own person, property or resources of the household. Because of the practice of demanding and giving dowry at the time of marriage of the girl to the husband's family, daughters are regarded as a loss to their parents' family. *Their labour and work whether productive or reproductive are socially devalued.* This inequity inherent in the social system is nurtured and perpetuated through a process of socialization. She not merely rationalizes but internalises this female status of disadvantage.

The Economic Dependence

The prohibitive cost to emergency intervention in labour, while women may even have no cash available in terms of seeking medicare in such emergency; this may be one of the causes for delay in seeking medicare and services. If community help is sought to reach the PHCs or Hospital, there were occasions, the women deposed before us, that community leaders might override even husband's wishes to save the woman from maternal mortality. Such incidents of community hold over individuals are experienced by villagers in Rajasthan and in Maharashtra tribal villages.

Socio-Economic Status of Women and Health

1. When Planners have allocated funds for BPL families, it is pathetic to find that it does not reach the beneficiaries for whom it is intended for. In Gurgaon in Haryana, when I was talking to the DRDA officials, I had occasion to personally watch how difficulties surface in deciding who a BPL is ? In spite of many possessing a BPL Card, so many questions were asked and many have been declared as not covered by the rules. Unless information about all dos and don'ts are given to them in advance, it cannot be expected of them to come prepared. All that those women knew was the card was their passport to the various provisions that they are entitled to. There has to be some mechanism helping them to correct the flaws and articulate their answers then and there. Many pregnant women go disheartened and not even understanding why their cards were not honoured ?

2. Poverty being the big issue and a disability, it complicates and compromises the health of the people, specially women and children. They though are covered under the below poverty line scheme, they were found caught up in the vicious cycle of lack of food, nutrition leading to anemia. Poor women were clamouring for jobs that can supplement their family income so that a little more can be put for child care and for their own well being.

3. Pregnancy and malnutrition being a deadly combination threatened many a lives and causing maternal deaths.

4. Economic causes shrouded in social ethos and cultural practices and vice versa. Which one takes priority over the other is hard to say. Poverty and lack of economic ability to buy food or access food leads to a variety of results adversely impacting on the health of people specially women and the girl child.

5. All these factors work simultaneously and thus the unbroken chain of causes emanating from the socio-economic determinants cannot be over ruled. "Girl children are under

nourished in their life cycle because of gender bias and poor food allocation, resulting in stunted growth leading to complications in pregnancy" (Royston 1989).

6. Women's contribution to national development and national productivity are not valued. Their economic dependency hampers their autonomy to seek medicare or institutional care in private hospital in whom they lay faith are costly. When we explained to the women that when they work in agricultural fields, the country gets food. The day the labour force will stop work, the country's "Food Basket" will become empty. They smiled but many did not understand the import of such a message.

7. In a nuclear family the woman is totally dependent on the husband and his income. But if she lives in a joint family where there are many hands who work and earn, sharing of better resources are possible. Though the women said they would love to have their independent homes, they said they still prefer to be in the joint families. They felt that it is better to have people at home who can mind the children when the women themselves are at work outside their homes.

8. Women of poorer households said that they were always on the look out for jobs so that they can earn and contribute to better care of their girl child.

9. Accessing institutional care even in emergencies is again a complex issue for women. She has to organize things at home for the family and her children and husband. Things are complicated for her since she has no freedom to think or decide. Every little act needs permission. There does not seem simple answers for her problems and needs.

10. Once she is allowed to seek institutional care, the lack of staff, supplies and equipment in the PHCs and sub-centres discourage women from accessing the same. The women prefer home delivery..

11. It is a welcome policy to train Anganwadi workers

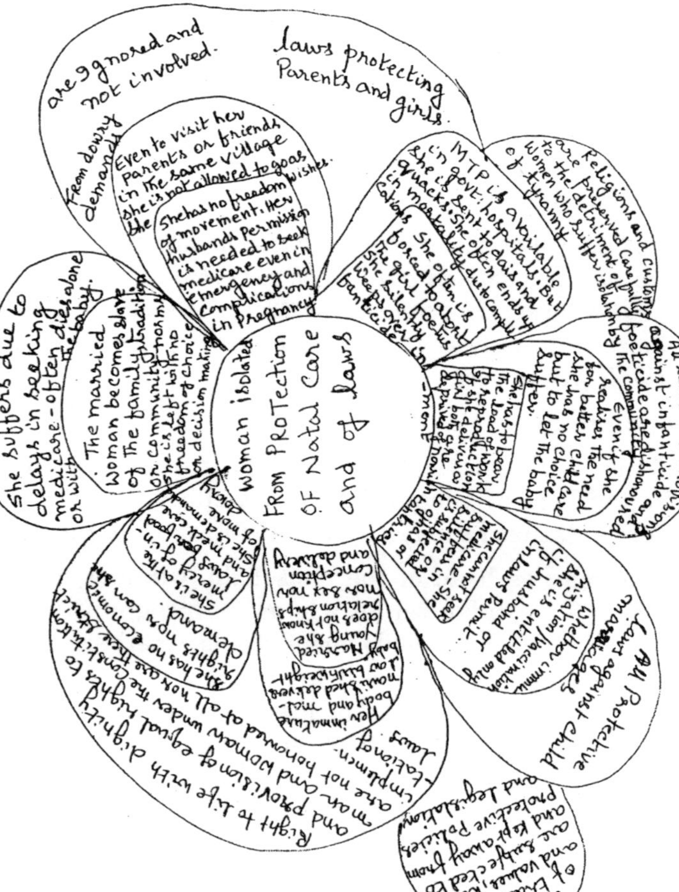
Woman isolated FROM PROTECTION OF Natal Care and of laws
are ignored and not involved.
laws protecting Parents and girls.
From dowry demands
Even to visit her parents or friends in the same village she is not allowed to go as she wishes.
She has no freedom of movement. Her husbands permission is needed to seek medicare even in emergency and complications in pregnancy
She suffers due to delays in seeking medicare - often dies alone or with the baby.
The married woman becomes slave of the family, tradition or community norms. She is left with no freedom of choice or decision making
MTP is available in govt. hospitals. But she is sent to dais and quacks. She often ends in mortality due to complications
All laws and provisions against infanticide and foeticide are dishonoured by the community.
Even if she realises the need for better child care she has no choice but to let the baby suffer.
Right to life with dignity and provision of equal rights to man and woman under the constitution are not honoured at all nor the implementation of laws.

as multiple workers including training in the basics of health and how to counsel women on safe motherhood and child care; also to handle medicines for cure for small ailments and to develop capacity to convince women on the values of iron and folic acid needed by pregnant and malnutritioned adolescents.

12. Even if medical services are offered free in the Primary and Sub-Health centres, sometimes the logistics are not women friendly. A close scrutiny of the above give us silent clues which may be relevant to the fine tuning of our existing policies. (we have touched upon them in our recommendations).

13. *Also just by erecting a basic health infrastructure in the village, women cannot be expected to rush to seek medical services. The complex system of village life does not promote easy access to any new structure even if it is available free of cost.*

Economic Status of the Family

This is a complicated issue covering many factors including lack of adequate health facilities, besides, the economic status of the family, impacting on IMR and MMR.

The man as head of the household, whether he is an employer or a labourer to whom the pregnant woman belongs, the woman's employment status, whether she is an earning member of the family are some of the attributes of the Socio-Economic status. The low economic value attached to girls along with the high economic liabilities with increasing demands of dowry at the time of marriage of the girls, put undue economic pressure on the household. To supplement family income, women seek paid work and become part of the informal and formal work force. Women though are paid much less than the men for equal jobs. Legislation provides equal pay for equal work similar jobs done by men. But the plight of women labour continues to suffer inequality in payments. It is common knowledge that domestic work done by women are not counted, nor valued as economic contribution to the household.

Medical and Non-Medical Factors Impact on MMR

Both medical and non-medical factors impact on maternal mortality.

MATERNAL DEATH: Is often not only a result of technical incompetence or medical negligence, but is also caused by superstitions and cultural practices Deliveries attended by traditional birth attendants; also lack of easy access to modern medicare due to lack of transportation facilities have also been quoted as of the contributing causes of MMR. Based on our field research, the points given below cover :

1. While reiterating that medical and non-medical factors influencing and impacting MMR; these are health behaviour: and actions people take or do not take for their health, e.g., attending or refusing to antenatal care by pregnant women or seeking help only when complications arise.

Our studies have shown when Kishori in Gujarghatal village in Rewari district of Haryana told that the Mother-in-law stopped her from attending to antenatal check ups and that she could not disobey her. In Renigunta of Chittoor district in Andhra Pradesh, Maya said that it is her husband's decision not allowing her to go in for antenatal. even when she was in advanced labour. In Khatawli village in Daru Heda Block PHC, when the pregnant woman's husband was away, it was the neighbours who had to take a decision to take Chaitri to the Health Centre. It was a case of breach and the foot of the baby was already out and the male child died after two hours after birth. Lack of autonomy for the woman and her dependency on the husband even at time of emergency has led to the death of the infant. And the woman started excessive bleeding. This could cause her death.

2. Reproductive behaviour that includes age at birth; pregnancy order and birth spacing and showing unwanted pregnancy, that carries stigma. Birth spacing is difficult for women since men refuse to adopt family procedures or take to contraceptives. This contributes to high fertility. Even when women are anemic and when the earlier child happens to be only 8 months old, they land up with another conception. Boori from village Akera in Haryana said that she has five girl children in a row and the mother-in-law insists as also the husband that she cannot take to family planning until such time she bears a male child. Who is concerned about her health? All they want is a male child.

3. Young women below the age of 18 years getting married, forced into conception within a year, face obstructed labour, because their body is not mature for motherhood and even child care. Death due to a number of biological factors occur. First child birth is risky for the adolescent mother and many cases of young mothers dying in maternity are many, though do not figure in the Census records.

In Tamil Nadu, in Madurai district, at Usilampatti village, the normal age of marriage is 14/15. Also these young girls are pressurized to conceive early. Many village women and the NGOs around informed us that early non-bearing of child is considered not merely a stigma but it psychologically affects the mother, when she is singled out, and jeered at, by all. In northern states stigma is attached to late conceptions.

4. Pregnancy order counts (parity) when women in their first pregnancy are likely to die than women having their second and third child. Again with the fourth child the risk rises. In Lonara in Nagpur district of Maharashtra and in Ambegaon in Nashik district of Maharashtra again, number of maternal deaths have occurred.

5. BIRTH SPACING: Many researches talk of the risk

of infant and child mortality due to birth spacing but ignore the impact on maternal mortality. For instance, in Harchandpura village of Bondse Block in Haryana, the woman refused antenatal care during all her four pregnancies and also ignored advice of the ANM to undergo sterilization. She was malnourished and there were very slim chances of her survival after the 5th child birth. Birth spacing does help the woman to recover from earlier child birth and recoup her strength. Birth spacing not only impacts on the infant, but helps maternal survival too.

6. Social pressure on women to bear male children. This boy preference, an ingrained socio-economic factor and forcing women to conceive again and again to try to bear a male baby may be a social requirement. But how about the woman's nutrition and health status. Not merely she is affected psychologically and emotionally, she has no value in the family until such time she bears a male child. Not merely this results in risk of survival to the mother but it leads to maternal mortality. Also the women whom we have met and spoken to also preferred male children to girl child. The perception that girl children are a liability has been the root cause of infanticides committed in Usilampatti in Tamil Nadu. Even today stray cases of infanticide are heard from Kallar community, a tribe who openly profess killing of their girl children.

7. The village view and social psyche are that girl child is a liability for life and that boys are income producers and also carriers of the family lineage.

Not only our research team interacted with Rajasthan women from Jaipur district and Jodhpur but also women from Tonk who they concede that they have to abort the female foetus because the innumerable problems the families have to face with a girl child. Therefore they marry their children young to avoid huge dowry and that they can absolve themselves of the girl's responsibility. When questioned if they die young in child birth how to save them, the women said, it is auspicious death if they die when their husbands are alive.

8. How is it that you women never go to the hospitals or primary health centres? They answered that they do not feel comfortable there. Hence they depend on the traditional dais at home; that is not only inexpensive; but also helps our belief in home deliveries and to get religious rituals performed by dais during and after delivery for a number of days.

It may be a surprise to many that in Tamil Nadu both in Madurai and in Salem districts, when the woman is pregnant, the family members approach the astrologers for "Jadakams" inquiring about the sex of the unborn and the prospects of survival of the mother. Their full faith in these predictors of their future, make them perform many pujas and rituals so that they can change the sex of the child in the womb. In tribal Andhra Pradesh, specially the women we have spoken to in Rangareddy district, they said they drink during pregnancy to make the foetus move actively; and they drink liquor after delivery to revive their lost strength. Their nutrition levels do not improve with drinks and the toxicants are harmful to the unborn too. Many foetus die in the womb and various crude ways of abortions end in maternal mortality.

Legally both foeticide and infanticide are banned and prohibited. But for the rural folk their beliefs and customary practices are the law. They are not merely ignorant and unaware of the duties imposed on citizens but social sanction is sacrosanct for them. Even threats of punishments are ignored. These strong socio-economic controls over people draws our attention for serious scrutiny and examination.

9. Unwanted pregnancies and resorting to abortions through dais and quacks lead to complications and maternal death.

Most of the unwanted pregnancies end up as abortions to get rid of the girl child in the foetus form. Even though the women have no decision making powers, even the husbands get ready to take them to quacks to get rid of unwanted pregnancies. Though the villagers by and large are illiterate, they come to know of the PNDT technology and approach abortion clinics which are surreptitiously run in the villages and towns. Except for the women of Tamil Nadu villages, all other states indulge in abortions. The Tamil Nadu women go for preventive action of going in for tubectomy after they are satisfied having two to three children. Haryana beats all, in illegal abortions because the Medical Termination of Pregnancy through MTP Clinics, Hospitals and Doctors have very little record of cases approaching them. For reasons of privacy and also to avoid embarrassment in public, and definitely to get rid of the prospects of a girl child, unwanted abortions take place in private Clinics. Illiteracy and ignorance do not seem to be any bar in accessing PNDT clinics and fraudulent persons parading as doctors.

Women approach these clinics at their advanced stages of pregnancy also. No government hospital will undertake such risks. And it is here, the private clinics make money, even at the risk of pushing woman to maternal mortality. Some cases were openly disclosed where some women who went for abortion came back as sterile women.

The Medical Termination of Pregnancy Act of 1971 has clearly provided abortion for women who are suffering from mental or physical problems due to unwanted pregnancies; where the growth of the foetus is stunted, where deformities are noticed in the foetus and where victims of rape do not want to continue with their pregnancies, women can opt for abortion in accredited hospitals, clinics and doctors. These certified hospitals and clinics and doctors keep regular registers of such cases that they have attended to. Unmarried girls and women also can seek access to such facilities. But the rural folk unaware of the safety net provided by this legislation and due to fear and apprehension of delays in government hospitals, they go to private clinics. These clinics and some of the private doctors take the risk of aborting even advanced pregnancies. The consequences are dangerous to the very life of women.

There are no records available of such abortions of unwanted pregnancies or and the outcome as maternal deaths. Husbands and mothers-in-law force the women to go for ultra sound tests to find out the sex of the foetus. If the unborn is identified as a female foetus, the women are pressurized physically, psychologically and emotionally to undergo abortions. Two women from the Rangareddy district confided that they had to go in for two abortions in a year. One can imagine the health and anaemic status of these women, and who belong to the BPL families. How can we reduce maternal mortality when such unhealthy practices are rampant, and unaccounted for. How can our Plans and Policies mitigate these complicated issues where women are entwined by the Socio-Cultural and Economic Compulsions ?

10. Our field staff could assess how complex a mixture it is, of the Socio-Economic and Cusltural Practices with Male Domination, conditioning the rural women to Complete Submission and Surrender. Women of Uttarakhand, unlike the rural women of other states did express their unhappiness over their plight as subjugated women.

11. Education of the mother has been emphasised by numerous researchers has a positive impact on the survival of women. But the villagers view education as a waste and unnecessarily time consuming. The girl child if she has survived has to mind her siblings and the older people at home; they have to tend to the cattle and work in the fields also. But in Haryana even the women who are matriculates are treated as any other uneducated ones. Uttarakhandis

most of their women are educated; but patriarchy has not left them free from its hold. But Tamil Nadu women though many of them are just neo-literates have asserted themselves to the extent that they insist on their daughters to be sent to school and that no one can stop them from getting tubectomy done as and when they wanted and also they are free to form themselves into Self Help Groups and generate some work and money. To some extent, one can admit that these Tamil Nadu women of the villages have partially succeeded in asserting their reproductive rights and of child care.

12. Irrespective of their State or the language group or to the caste to which they belonged, women unanimously agreed that their lives are tied up in too many knots and it is impossible to be free from them. They said they respect their community beliefs and some of the practices. But when it affects their daughters, they were extremely unhappy. They wanted their daughters to be educated.

13. NO MOTHER WOULD LIKE TO KILL HER OWN CHILD: In Magudanchavadi village in Salem district in Tamil Nadu, our field staff, spoke to the SHGs who got a mother-in-law arrested for committing infanticide of her grand daughter in the presence of the baby's mother, (her daughter-in-law.) The baby's mother cited how her baby was strangulated. It was heart rending to hear the same said our team members. Women, once they are informed they could organize themselves into groups, the NGOs did a good job in training them in self-confidence and made them aware of their rights and duties. But similar infanticide was committed in the PHC premises in Daru Heda block. When the doctor and the midwife went out to wash their hands, in a matter of minutes, the newly born healthy girl child was found dead. The mother of the child after delivery-fatigue was sleeping. No eye witness was there to complain. The case was not pursued. On questioning the mother-in-

law who feigned ignorance of what ever happened. The constant presence of the NGOs in the village and because of the regular training programmes they conduct and encourage women to be self-confident and self-supporting have really brought change in their attitudes and behaviour.

High fertility means higher risk of maternal mortality. The risk of MMR after the birth of the third child is high. The fear that infertility would lead to divorce and even husband's threat to go in for bigamous marriage and polygamous marriages keep women captive in pregnancies. This is thought of as safeguard against those eventualities.

Empirical evidence show that illiterate women have high rates of fertility than the educated ones. This though true in all the States except in Haryana, where even 10th class pass women's fertility levels are as high due to compelling acceptance of their husband's dictates.

It is another story about the Uttarakhand women. While men go away to the plains in search of jobs, the women belonging to the labour class are almost kept in continuous state of pregnancy. This is thought of as safeguard against women going astray or getting exploited by other men. As a single parent the pregnant woman works hard, going long distances, fetching water, fuel and attending to the household chores and taking care of their children etc. Kumaoni women start working after the 22nd day after delivery. Many of them confided to our research team, women suffer from prolapse of their uterus. Without medical attention, many of them contract infections and even cancer resulting in death.

14. The Headmaster of Primary School Akera as also the Doctor of Daru Heda Primary Health Centre Haryana suggested a remedial measure that will have the highest and maximum impact on fertility and survival of the pregnant women and prevent maternal mortality: That is by reducing the rate of girl child drop out from schools and educating

them further.. Investment in education thus has been over emphasized as the best way to reduce fertility and to cut short the consequent chain of debility syndrome among women leading to death. This impact process through education may seem remote but it is a long lasting cure to eradicate irrational and deep rooted socio-economic beliefs and determinants that cause both maternal and infant mortality. In village Bamdoli in Gurgaon district of Haryana, school going girls requested us to talk to their fathers to send them for higher education because, the fathers want their young daughters to get married even though they are below 17 years (then). Educated girls will naturally raise their marriageable age in order to pursue education and this will be of immense impact on the mothers to be and their health and survival. But the parents specially fathers say that girls are Paraya- *dhan* and they ask, 'why to keep them for long'. Also it is risky to keep young girls at home if unmarried.

15. All these views expressed by women and opinions of parents and suggestions made by the school master and the doctor to contain drop out rates of girls from schools show, how the symptoms of the socio-economic malaise, are overlooked as part of village life style and the cultural grip over people and specially women, continue. The dangerous socio-economic factors determine and affect almost all aspects of a woman, throughout her life cycle.

16. We questioned women in many of the villages we surveyed as how they passively abet the killing of the girl child either by the dai or by the grand mother. Their answer was that, bearing a girl child reduces their status in the family. That they cannot overrule the decision taken by their elders. They said that, family honour has to be guarded even if it meant sacrificing their girl child. They added, "after all we cannot expose our own people and we have to respect our elders for whatever they do". Again to our teams question, "how is it they do not rebel against their husbands

domination over all of their actions, they said, 'no' and added, "after all man is the head of the family; We must listen to him. How can we question him ?"

Reproductive Decision Making

Women's control over there own sexuality and reproductive decision making is constantly affected by a range of forces as mentioned before, mainly due to lack of empowerment of women. The household and the community pressure on the women to bear many children (high fertility) closely relate to the village concept of economic and social security by bearing male children and gain status and respect in the household and the community. Also, son preference relates to lineage and inheritance to property rights or resources of the parents. Social and economic constraints coupled with cultural practices and maternal factors named socio-demographic causes all put together have reduced the woman to a servile status where her life is constantly threatened.

Reproductive decision making is almost nil on the part of the village woman contained by social values: Cultural practices leave no room for woman's freedom and decision making. Independence is almost a misnomer. Crippled by numerous constraints, woman is bereft of her own reproductive rights. A few women from Uttarakhand and strangely from Rajasthan also, dared to share with our team of researchers that, "they feel that they need to be treated better by her husbands and their mothers-in-law.

Having got used to this low profile, women with their own low esteem, do not consider their discomfort in their physique as worthy of complaint. Domestic violence adds to the sense of low esteem. To avoid any embarrassment to the family, the women suffer deprivations in silence. It may be too late when they openly seek medicare for their wounds due to violence perpetrated on them. Even when the family realizes the impending threat of complications in pregnancy, they hesitate to seek medical assistance for the pregnant woman. This is also due to their community's perception of modern medi-care, and fear of the police case in case if they found wounds on the body of the woman. Though ignorant of the laws, the villagers are afraid of the police that they may be arrested and put in jail. One graduate woman in Hamirpur village of Haryana and a village woman from Nakkalpatti in Tamil Nadu questioned, "why not? After all our husbands have a right to bash us when we do; things without their permission". Where is 'empowerment' when women themselves do not want it ?

EDUCATION : A POSITIVE IMPACT ON INFANT SURVIVAL AND MATERNAL HEALTH

Education positively impacts on reducing maternal mortality and infant mortality in a number of different ways :-

1. In lowering fertility: With less number of pregnancies: women can deliver less number of children and thus reducing the risk of mortality.
2. Women's social status and self image get increased by education.
3. Help delay in early marriage and thus late child bearing.
4. Educated women can understand the anatomy of the body and physiology of reproduction.
5. Disposed to accept complications and risks in pregnancy.
6. Can opt for modern medication and refuse fatalism and superstitious practices.
7. Understand best child care practices.
8. Will be willing to convince their husbands on family planning methods.
9. Less likely to accept dangerous practices during pregnancy and after delivery.
10. Women's education helps better employment

prospects.

11. Education influences quality of performance and can demand equal pay.
12. The nature and type of employment can help limit fertility.
13. Educated women can realize the harmful effects of heavy workload during pregnancy and after delivery.
14. Understands the need for rest for three months before delivery.
15. Can convince family members of the need for institutional health care; Can avoid seeking delays in institutional health care.
16. She can and will be able to prevent infant and maternal mortality.
17. She can convince other women on advantages of seeking institutional health care.
18. Will be aware of safe motherhood practices; and avoid illegal abortions.
19. Can realize legal limitations to child and adolescent marriages and dowry demands.
20. Educated women can assert physical and social mobility.
21. Educated women can convince all and send girls to schools.

To sum up, an educated mother is an insurance against maternal and infant mortality. Where women's decision making capacity is denied by household and community power relations, maternal education helps to increase awareness to the need to seek medical intervention in emergencies. This will clearly be sufficient to increase their use of health services. Education can be a true aid in helping better implementation of governmental policies and programmes as also to assert themselves to think and act.

Education alone can free them from the grip of irrational beliefs, inhuman practices and the Socio-Economic-Cultural Factors that have been reducing women to demonizing levels.

Areas where low female literacy rates are, areas where the fewest births are attended to by trained personnel. Garhwali women with whom we have long hours of conversation, majority of them are literate said that they had to reconcile to the hard labour they had to bear with because of the geography of the area. This they said is inescapable for them to walk long distances and fetch fuel and water. They did regret their high fertility rate since their husbands refuse, use of contraceptives or other family planning me thods. Though governments offer Rs.1000 and more for men opting to undergo family planning operations, there are no takers not because of men's refusal but mainly because the women fear that their men will go weak with the operation, though it is very simple.

Another problem the Uttarakhand women face is that the health centres and hospitals have no doctors nor the required equipment or medicines for deliveries and operations. Since most of them are educated they are questioning why such neglect is prevailing in the health service delivery system? Due to these drawbacks, women's survival is not still certain in these parts.

RITUALS ENDANGERING WOMEN'S LIVES

Religious rituals are performed in order to assist the woman in labour. But it is only the traditional birth attendant who is asked by the family to perform these rituals. Pregnancy being considered 'impure', only this low caste Dai is allowed to do whatever has to be done. The woman who delivered is treated as an untouchable and no one is allowed to go to her room where she is cutting the umbilical cord and examination of the vagina, removal of the placenta are treated as rituals that the Dai has to perform. In other states, it is the mother who has the first right to cut the umbilical cord. Dais are not aware of hygiene or aseptic practices and techniques. They even fail to wash their hands and the instruments if any. Unclean objects are used during vaginal examination and in cutting the cord. This leads to urinary infection, tetanus, genital infection and sepsis thereby putting women at risk of death and maternal mortality. *Treatment of obstructed labour by untrained Dais is often dangerous. Herbal medicines are given for better contraction during labour. This is widely reported to cause uterine rupture.* Our surveys recorded such occurrences in Umrale village in Nashik and in Lonara village in Nagpur district of Maharashtra, remote Rethoj and Harchandpur villages in Haryana, Nauta in Chamoli district of Uttarakhand. Insertion of caustic substances into the vagina of the delivered woman to restore it to normal vaginal conditions are other purification techniques adopted by the Dais. The doctors in the primary health centres reacted vehemently and called them utterly dangerous practices that definitely lead to maternal mortality. Also washing the baby with cow dung, putting cowdung at the cut edge of the umbilical cord and rub the child with red mud are other rituals that the Uttarakhandi villagers practice. Sprinkling of cow urine after the mother is given a bath with scalding hot water, with curds and other elements thrown into it is another ritual. One cannot find scientific significance to these practices.

Food Taboos

Pregnant women are expected to make dietary changes that reduce their intake of foods high in protein, in calcium, milk and green vegetables. These are forbidden in many rural societies for reasons that the foetus is located in the stomache and that it may grow enormous. Thus pregnant woman receives fewer calories than what she is normally expected of to fully feed herself and the baby in the womb. Though massive intake of sodium is permitted by the traditional rural folk. While the Kumaonis have definite list of prohibited for women during menstruation, in pregnancy and after delivery, even water is amongst the list of things not to be taken. In Haryana the quantity of food intake during pregnancy is slashed fearing the unborn will grow big resulting in difficult delivery. Rajasthan women are fed with methi, ajwain and hing to keep the stomach clear of flatulence. Harchandpur village women of Haryana said that ajwain if given, the 'booth' will stick to the body and will not leave; while people in other villages in Haryana said, 'when ajwain is given to pregnant women, some persons have to be posted to guard her".

In contrast in Tamil Nadu villages, where we actually happen to be present during one of the celebrations done at 6 months of the first pregnancy of a woman. Many village women came with tasty sweetmeats for the pregnant woman to eat. Others decked her with bangles and lot of flowers. She was made to feel like a queen. This is a celebration for motherhood. The Tamil women believed that what ever the pregnant woman wishes to eat has to be given even if it is in the late hours of the night. Of course the prohibited foods are papaya, and some of the gas producing vegetables.

Stranger still is the stories of Andhra tribal women, who drink during pregnancy. In Rangareddy district they told us that drinks will help the foetus to move freely in the stomach, and which is necessary for its proper growth. They also have no concept of nutrition or iron or folic acid nor understanding of their need for pregnant women. After delivery, alcoholic drink they believe is a must for the lactating mother to recoup her strength. The only taboo they follow is giving up 'beedi' smoking during pregnancy. But the tribal women of Maharashtra take to alovera that is available in the form of cactus all over in those dry areas.

Our team of surveyors exclaimed that, "India is an anthropological wonder". Too many beliefs and numerous practices. Which one is right or bad is hard to say.

The one common factor that threads all the villages is

male domination over women, absence of faith in modern medication and medicines and above all women's lack of empowerment and many ending up with maternal mortality. This they would rather attribute to fate or punishment given by the spirits for wrongs committed by woman either in this life now or in the past, 'janam'. Besides tampering with the health and well being of the pregnant woman, by these numerous practices, the unborn and the newborn infants get to be more vulnerable to infant mortality.

Villagers averse to Institutional Deliveries : Pre-Sex Determination Tests Welcome

Literacy and education may not be priorities in these villages of Rajasthan, Haryana, Maharashtra and Andhra Pradesh, specially for the girls. But even the ignorant knows about Ultrasound Tests and the technology available to detect and reveal the sex of the unborn foetus. The law pertaining to prenatal diagnostics techniques (Prohibition of Misuse and Regulation) Act as amended as on today, restricts and prohibits the use of ultrasound tests for disclosing the sex of the foetus. Private clinics surreptitiously revealing the sex of the foetus and are minting money; they are commercial shops who are unconcerned about the diminishing sex-ratio of girls versus boys. These tests instead of helping people to come to know of any deformities in the growth of the unborn, they are focusing on the sex of the foetus. The rush to these centres end up with women rushing to abortion dens run by compounders and mechanics who parade as practising doctors. Otherwise the village women run to the traditional dais or quacks who create complications and resulting in women's death. These illegal clinics take the risk of aborting pregnancies even at advanced stages lending both the child in the womb and the mother to death.

There is no count of these illegal abortions because no one keeps a record of the same. Governmental enforcement machinery took strong steps to close such clinics who violate the legal prescriptions. However, the village women in Rethoj told our team of researchers that these ultra sound machines are some times stacked in the fields to avoid action by the enforcement. Though the women do not openly disclose as to where they had abortions, they did share with us that they had to abort the girl child.

Many women belonging to different States, who deposed before us, strongly felt that if unwanted pregnancies could be eliminated, fertility could drop to replacement levels. As per UNICEF, sources 2001, Indian women numbering 100,000 die of pregnancy related causes every year, which is about 18% of total global maternal deaths in addition many women are disabled by complications of pregnancy, abortions and child birth. There is no data available on the number of abortions. Only a very few done as medical termination of pregnancy cases in accredited hospitals here and there may be the only data in the records. Most of the abortions are illicit and done through dais and quacks which have no count at all, many of them end in maternal mortality. These practices add to further difficulties in collecting the data as also assessing their impact on maternal survival and maternal death.

Though very few cases surface, it is relevant to quote the case of Dr. Jacob George vs. State of Kerala, 1994 AIR SCW 2282, CRL APP R (SC) 214: 1994. Death while causing miscarriage an accused homeopath doctor, caused death to the deceased while operating not for any permissible causes, the Court held the accused liable to conviction under Section 314 IPC. The convict was ordered to pay Rupees one lakh to the child left behind by the deceased. Even the Sample Registration Survey (SRS) declared that there are no available data on illegal abortions or on foeticide. Thus the count of maternal mortality rates are very much under estimates.

A positive trend we found was in Tamil Nadu where a growing number of village women in Tamil Nadu were opting for family planning procedures after having two or three children. It is a welcome change. This practice of seeking institutional services is contributing to reduction in maternal mortality. Earlier illegal abortions also went under cover of miscarriages and physical deformities of the foetus etc.

Through the PNDT Act, the government sought to arrest the growing undergrowth and deformities of the foetus and not to be misused or intended to reveal the sex of the foetus. But this policy has almost failed. Instead Fast Reduction of Sex Ratio of Girls vis a vis Boys is accelerated by the Prenatal Diagnostic techniques tests conducted by private medical practitioners and clinics.

The State of Haryana tops the list of PNDT Test users and a number of clinics are conducting these tests. This practice of going in for tests reinforce their son preference. It has definite impact on female mortality and female sex-ratio.

Beliefs and cultural practices detrimental to the health of the girl child and woman: In the states of Tamil Nadu, Haryana and Rajasthan, people in villages carry on with the myth that girls are liabilities and are meant to be married young and sent away to their in-laws family. Thus the child marriages are rampant as sickness. When I was in the National Commission for Women, I could conduct the first investigation of the Saathin's case from Bateri village of Jaipur district, of Rajasthan. In due performance of her duties, the Saathin tried to persuade families in the village to stop child marriages. She instead became a victim for trying to uphold the State law and State policy prohibiting child marriages. Even the judiciary in Rajasthan could not rise high above the caste bias as they did in the famous case of Bhanwari Bai, a Saathin. She only had appealed to villagers not to conduct or solemnize child marriages. She was gang raped by those who conducted child marriages in their homes. The little said of Rajasthan the better, when enmasse child marriages are conducted during Akha Teej, the government looks the other way. In spite of the political complexion of the day, no one would like to touch these sensitive issues lest the political aspirants and politicians may lose votes in elections.

The key question arises here as to what should we call it—a superstition, a myth, turned into a hardened practice or is it an economic determinant or a feature which militates against the law of the State namely the Child Marriage Prohibition Act which lies in the shelves of the lawyers and Courts. States do not want to touch this issue because of' Electoral politics'.

The feed back received from our Surveyors in Tamil Nadu shows a new trend of putting an end to infanticide. In Salem district, it has been a cruel practice of killing the new born girl for fear of dowry demand made at the girl's marriage. The wrong belief although exists that boys alone are considered as caretakers of the parents in their old age and can perform the last rites after their death.

It may be relevant to talk of the diehard practices like Satipratha that has taken away innocent lives. Though law has banned such inhuman practices, no one seems to be afraid of the law nor honour the law. Social sanction still exists for such customs. Even judiciary in Daurala case where a young widow was drugged and coaxed to sit on the pyre of her dead husband to commit sati. Thousands of onlookers were witness to the incident but the Court did not convict any for want of proof. Whether to call the legal system as ineffective or biased, is hard to say. *But this reveals the stronghold of custom and practices on the rural folk and in this particular case the judiciary also. Such similar incident occurred in Madhya Pradesh in 2004. Even after passing legislations to combat evil practices we are not able to eliminate inhuman practices like Sati, dowry burning, infanticide and foeticide? These cases only prove how in the name of custom, tradition and superstition, negative practices are nurtured by society for generations. This is ample evidence to show how deep seated superstitious practices are directly and indirectly leading to infant mortality and maternal mortality. Such are the causes that contribute to the slow pace of reduction in maternal mortality.*

Gender Violence and Maternal Mortality

The issue of violence is to be firmly placed on the health agenda. Woman battered during pregnancy is twice likely to miscarriage and four times more likely to have a low birth weight baby than those who are not beaten. It has grave impact on malnourished women. Gender violence is amongst one of the significant causes of morbidity and maternal mortality. *Safe motherhood initiatives remain limited to the notion of reproductive health; there is danger of ignoring the importance of women's emotional, physical well being which are beyond reproductive autonomy (Heise 1993).*

Family planning though needed to stabilize population, and help better spacing of children, it is definitely not the concern of the village men living with their own beliefs and practices. The village women in Hamirpur in Haryana, Usalimpatti in Madurai and in Rangareddyin Andhra Pradesh, Nandaprayag in Uttarakhand, Bateri village in Jaipur - Rajasthan and Nashik in Maharashtra equivocally said that it is their husbands who object to the use of contraceptives. With early marriages of young girls, males could control female sexuality and support higher fertility. Also lack of communication between husband and wife on matters of sexuality and the age old practice of holding male dominance in the household prevails.

Why Women Resist to Seek Medi-Care : Social and Physical Distance Big Barrier

Many of the women in groups, interviewed in the villages, have given a number of reasons for not able to access medical services through institutional health care. They are :

1. The fear that hospital staff may ridicule the tradition and practices of a community and impose unfamiliar food to eat. Because the mother after delivery is given almost nothing but black tea with only a pinch of milk at home.
2. Sloping posture for delivery by village women is not appreciated.
3. They feel that the dress they are asked to wear in the hospital is culturally inappropriate. Women prefer to opt to deliver in a known and sympathetic surrounding outside the health centres. (Prevention of maternal mortality network, 1992).
4. Cultural misunderstanding, lack of sensibility among health professionals can lead to a breakdown in communications between women and health workers, which is not conducive to high quality of care. Women in Kwedal Kumaon and Nauta in Garhwal from Tonk in Rajasthan started gigling on hearing the same.
5. Women prefer home deliveries attended by dais, in their familiar habitat.
6. Operations of any kind are dismissed and stigmatized in their village community.
7. The irrational belief may be such that if a woman does not deliver normally, she is thought of to have failed in her essential role as a wife. Our findings are with a dai attending at home things would be better.
8. These may contribute to the, "social distance and causes" for village women, in accessing health services.
9. Other main reason in the Indian context rooted in strictures against contact with male health personnel.

10. Village Women from Uttarkhand, Rajasthan and Andhra Pradesh openly said maternal and child health staff, must be all women. This is a pre-requisite to expect women coming for institutional care for deliveries.
11. Poor quality of antenatal care and screening, discourage women from attending these facilities.
12. Delays in diagnostic treatment with decisions to go for c-section may also lead to fatal consequences.
13. Maternal health care should not be dehumanizing. A patient should be treated with respect and compassion by the health personnel. Unfortunately such expectations are not fulfilled. On the contrary, *the women's groups with whom we had long many hours of discussion stated that the governments, original recognition of, "the mutuality of the rights of the child and mother is a direct response to the implications of maternal mortality and maternal morbidity"*. (Nurske 1991).
14. *Child survival has a bearing on mother's rights and vice-versa. Reducing maternal mortality is an appropriate measure to diminish infant and child mortality. Art. 24 of the UN convention on the Rights of the Child relates to maternal mortality in para 3, "all State parties shall take all effective and appropriate measures with a view to abolishing traditional practices prejudicial to the health of the children." Therefore legal and international commitments to child rights, child's physical, mental and spiritual and right of social development can be important in tackling factors affecting maternal mortality. But how do we expect an ANM and an Anganwadi worker or even ASHA to know about these international commitments?*

15. *Generally, the villagers do not consider government hospitals as helpful care takers. Though they prefer hospitals to the primary health centres. The delays in government hospitals discourage women to approach them. Besides, many village women regretted that, "the first thing the doctors ask us to get an ultrasound test done.* The cost and the delays involved discourages women to approach the government hospitals. They said they prefer to go to the private ones if they can afford or go back to their dais at the time of delivery".

A wlecome experiment amidst the gloomy environment of maternal mortality and infant mortality has been the combined work culture practised by the Anganwadi worker and the ANM from the Primary Health Centre at the village level. Mutually linked child survival and safe motherhood, both find a place in a synthesized government project i.e. the integrated child development scheme. It is here in this infrastructure, is incorporated both child's and mother's basic need for nutrition. This infrastructure is meant to attend to pregnant and lactating mothers besides children. Their joint role of synthesizing the ICDS with the Health service delivery system (through the Community Health Centre, Primary Health Centres and Sub-health Centres) are expected to show signs of success.

4

LACK OF EMPOWERMENT OF WOMEN A MAJOR CONSTRAINT

What is Empowerment?

- Right to life with dignity.
- Right to equality and equal treatment.
- Right to be loved.
- Right to decide ones Right.
- Right to pursue education.
- Right to seek health care.
- Right to clean environment.
- Right to invoke the laws.
- Right to share family resources.
- Right to decide when to marry.
- Right to decide when to be a mother.
- Has a right to nutritious food and good health.
- Right to family planning.
- Right to shelter.
- Right to livelihood.
- Right to economic independence.
- Right to work outside home.
- Right to share in parental property.
- Right to resist violence.
- Right to refuse cultural practices and taboos.

- Right to equal wages.
- Right to minimum wages.
- Right to support services from NGOs/Voluntary Organisations.
- Right to political participation.
- Right to vote in elections.
- Right to attend gram sabha meetings.
- Right to information.
- Right to free expression.
- Right to safety.

The lack of empowerment of women thrives in a social environment where derogatory practices like foeticide, infanticide, child marriages, dowry demands, violence on women and the girl child, sexual abuse of women and the girls, where exploitation both economic, social and religious are perpetrated; Where rule of law is ignored and disregarded, and above all, where the women are discriminated and their human rights are flouted, both at home and in the society. The empowerment of women becomes a very big condition to diminish infant mortality rates and the maternal mortality rates which in our country still persist and is not showing any speedy decline.

Why this Pathetic Situation is Continuing in Our Country?

The answer lies in the fact that both men and women are socialized in patriarchical norms and these values are nurtured for generations. But families who have chosen the path of education, developed rationality and a scientific temper, have realized their potential and have some protection from the laws that exist to protect them from all violations.

However, in a village situation, even today woman has a subservient role to play both at home, at work place and

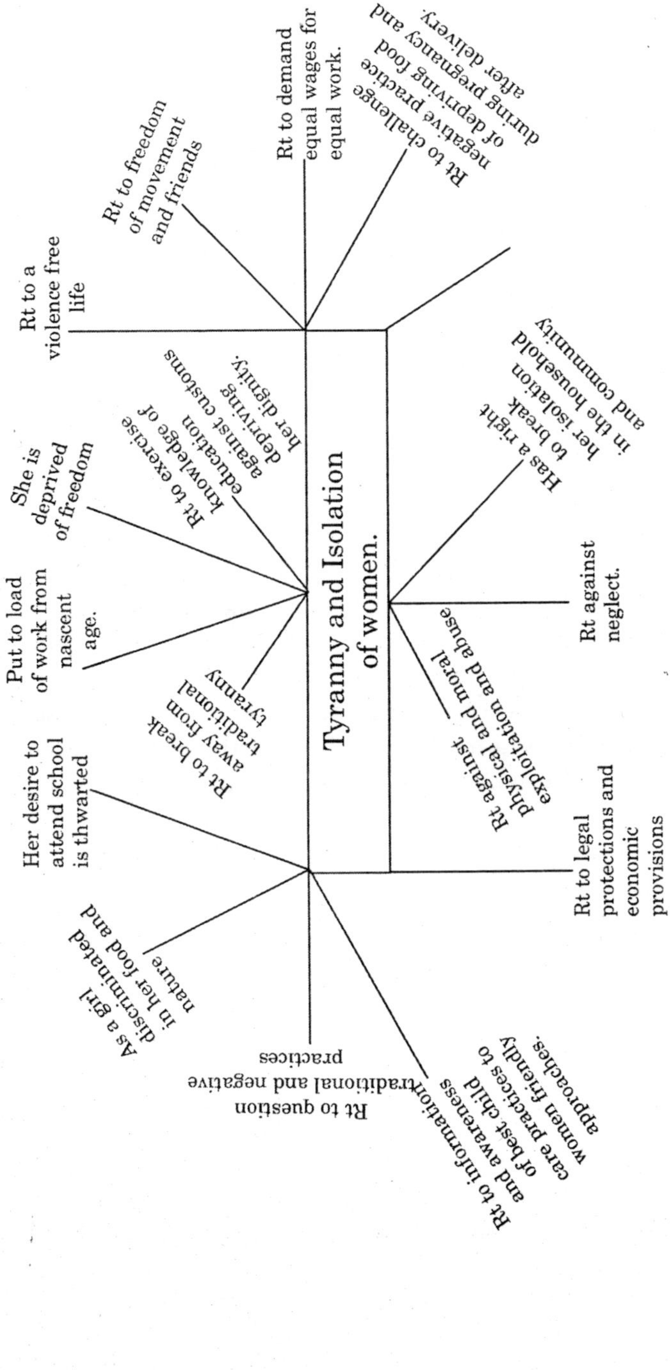
Tyranny and Isolation of women.
Rt to a violence free life
Rt to freedom of movement and friends
Rt to demand equal wages for equal work.
Rt to challenge negative practice of depriving food during pregnancy and after delivery.
She is deprived of freedom
Rt to exercise knowledge of education against customs depriving her dignity.
Put to load of work from nascent age.
Rt to break away from traditional tyranny
Her desire to attend school is thwarted
As a girl discriminated in her food and nature
Rt to question traditional and negative practices
Rt to information and awareness of best child care practices to women friendly approaches.
Has a right to break her isolation in the household and community
Rt against neglect.
Rt against physical and moral exploitation and abuse
Rt to legal protections and economic provisions

in the community. She has no freedom of choice; From her growing days she foregoes the right to pursue what she wanted, whether to refuse early marriage and thus early motherhood, whether to shun the greedy groom who demands dowry, whether to decide the number of children she would like to produce, whether she can pursuade her husband to use the family planning devices, whether to seek health care in the primary health centre, or, whether to have a share in the household resources, whether to decide to send her children to school, specially the girl children, and above all, whether she has the freedom of movement in the village and liberty to spend her meager means on herself and her children.

The empowerment of women can remove gender disparities that manifest in various forms; the most obvious being the trend of declining female "Sex-Ratio" in the population for the last two decades:

The underlying causes of gender inequalities are related to socio-economic structure, which is based on informal and formal norms and socio-cultural practices. Women, particularly those belonging to weaker sections of society, majority of whom are in the rural areas, are in the unorganised sector. Their access to education, health and productive resources among others is inadequate. Therefore, they remain largely marginalised, poor and socially excluded.

The empowerment is an all emcompassing concept wherein a woman can exert her freedom to take decisions concerning her health, her reproductive health rights, social behaviour and her child care needs. The ability to pursue vocations of her choice and be free to educate her children specially the girl children, too becomes a close possibility.

Once empowered she has a right to refuse practices that are derogative to her and her children, e.g. keeping girl child away from school and play, getting her to marry in her adoloscent age or pushing her to conceive early and the family members, greed to expect only a male child. Practising traditional food practices leading her girl child to abject malnutrition. And instead the mother can give nourishing diet that will be beneficial to her and her children's growth and well being. To take a simple example, an empowered woman can resume breastfeeding of the child immediately after delivery as advised by the doctors and an act not unoften prohibited in lakhs of Indian villages.

In short, once she understands, that no one other than her has a right to deprive her of her human rights to life with dignity and be not subjected to indignities or suffer domestic violence on her or on her children, she can to some degree escape distress and destitution in her life. Even though the laws the land has endowed her with equal protection against discrimination, seldom every one obeys the laws.

Lack of empowerment breeds other ills. Being an illiterate and illinformed woman, she is subjected to her socio-economic and family imposed cultural constraints. She having internalized her socialization of women's secondary role in the household, in the community and the world at large, continues to suffer even though she cries for her rights to empowerment. This distorted self esteem is not merely the creation of her imagination or illusion. It is thrust on her in the name of custom, tradition and allied practice and expected of her role as a son producing machine. One can safely term it as superstitious belief that she attributes all her ills to her fate instead of realizing that it is the male psyche of dominance nurtured for generations that she suffers the tragedy of both IMR and of MMR.

Some Helpful Efforts

The mother and child health programme as it has been

evolved in the years highlights how changes have been effected from time to time, by government making efforts to design the programmes to help women and children at the rural Ievel. The milestones are:

1. YEAR 1952	Family Planning programme adopted by Govt. of India.
2. YEAR 1961	Dept. of Family Planning created in Ministry of Health.
3. YEAR 1971	Medical termination of pregnancy act (MTP) Act.
4. YEAR 1977	Renaming of family planning to Family Welfare.
5. YEAR 1978	Expanded programme on Immunization (EP).
6. YEAR 1985	Universal immunization programme + National Oral Rehydration Therapy (ORT) Programme.
7. YEAR 1992	Child survival and safe motherhood programme (CSSM).
8. YEAR 1996	Target free approach.
9. YEAR 1997	Reproductive and Child Health Programme - 1 : (RCH-I).
10. YEAR 2005	Reproductive and Child Health Programme - 2 : (RCH-II).

The National Health Policy 2002 and Vision 2020 India were directed to minimize the regional variations in the areas of RCH and population stabilization through an integrated, focussed, participatory programme; it was to meet the unmet demands of the population to get an assured and equitable quality services. The five year phase of RCH II, was launched in 2005, with a vision to bring about outcomes as envisioned, integral to the Millennium Development goals, the National Population Policy 2000 and the Tenth Five Year Plan.

Sadly though none of the targets of major policies and goals for the Tenth Five Year Plan (2002-2007) could be achieved: The details given below show the unachieved goals:

Indicators	*10th Plan Goals 2002-2007*	*RCH II Goals (2005-2010)*	*National Population Policy 2005-2010*	*Millennium Development Goals 2000-2015*
Population growth	16.2% 2001-2011	16.2% 2001-2011	—	—
Infant mortality rate	45/1000	35/1000	30/1000	—
Maternal mortality rate	200/100,000	100/100,000	100/100,000	Reduced by/from 1990 level
Total fertility Rate	2.3	2.11	2.1	—
Couple protection rate	65%	65%	Meet 100% needs	—

A summarized view that emerges here is as given below:

What is lack of empowerment?

- Right not assured.
- Discriminated at every step.
- Reduces her to low status and loaded with work.
- No right to take decision.
- No right to pursue education/or late marriage.
- No right to decide the size of her family.
- Lacks nutrition.
- Lacks good food.
- Lacks right to seek health care even in emergency.

- Deprived of sanitation.
- No Hygiene nor potable water.
- No idea of sterilisation.
- Low status for delivering girl child.
- Tradition-culture bound.
- No right to breastfeed her child immediately after delivery.
- Half fed in pregnancy.
- Is malnutritioned.
- Hard work in her daily life.
- Lack of resources.
- Lacks property rights.
- No right of mobility.
- No right in family resources.
- No education.
- No concept of good health.
- No right to demand.
- Ignorant of laws.
- No idea and right to childcare.
- No right to take decisions about her children.
- Lack of opportunity to employment.
- Lacks equal pay for equal work.
- Socialised with belief in Evil Spirits, sorcery, witches.
- Lacks right to resist abuse of her children.
- Lacks ability to feed her children.
- Lacks empowerment.
- No continuous voluntary support available.
- Lives in hostile surroundings lacks protection against abuse.

Rural Woman is kept tradition bound against her life and liberty.	Woman is not considered as having any health problems.	She cannot resist the cultural practice of applying cowdung on the edge of umbilical cord of the baby	She is loaded with household chores even during pregnancy and even immediately after delivery	New born is branded with hot object all over the body as a cure.
She has no say in household issues or about her Children's well being.	She is married young by giving dowry to the in-laws.	She is forced to conceive early after marriage.	Process of child birth is considered as pollution.	Only pregnancy and delivery are noticed and a untrained dai alone is to handle deliveries.

WOMEN'S LACK OF EMPOWERMENT ACCELERATES IMR & MMR

She is considered a reproductive machine	She is kept in unhygienic space during delivery and dirty rays are used for her and her baby	She has no right to feed her baby for days.	After delivery she is hungry but is given only dark tea and no-nutrition. This again is a cultural practice.	Until she delivers a boy she cannot opt for sterilisation or family planning
She is not to decide how many children she wants and conceive	She is looked down upon for bearing a girl child. She is respected only if she delivers a male child.	She is socialised into submission and nurtures low esteem including that of her girl child.	Husband is the decision maker along with his parents.	There is no concept of her morbidity levels.

Select Ground Reality of Constraints and Determinants to be altered would be as given below:

- Woman is a bundle of duties.
- With no rights.
- Village woman has no social or legal persona.
- She cannot cook what she wants without permission.
- She has no right to mobility.
- Custom, cultural practice govern all her life.
- No right to take any decision on family issues.
- She has no right to refuse to work, or follow tradition, or husband's dictats.
- Only traditional dai can attend to her delivery.
- Cannot refuse branding on child with hot iron or needle as cure.
- Lacks nutrition, child care.
- She abets murder of her girl child by dai/in-laws.
- She has no voice against abuse, violence and exploitation.
- She can't say no to cow dung application to baby's umbilical cord.
- She cannot invoke laws.
- She has no means of protection.
- A total life of dependency.
- If belongs to SC/ST/OBC
- Lacks equal treatment
- By authorities.

To sum up, one can candidly assert even today the lack of empowerment of women has increased the incidence of infant mortality and maternal mortality? The numerous disabilities that a woman suffers and experiences directly and indirectly influences the stagnating and undiminishing infant mortality and maternal mortality.

The mutuality of relationship and inter-relatedness of the mother and the child is affected in a number of ways by lack of empowerment of women.

The child's total dependence on the mother from its survival, to growth without disease and debility is common knowledge. But in the name of custom, tradition and cultural practices, this mutual maternal and child oneness is interfered with and heavily impacted on their chances of survival. From the day the child is conceived in the womb, its proper growth depends on its nurture through the mother. But where is the nurture? The so-called cultural practice is depriving the nourishment needed for the child and the mother. Even before birth, the health of the unborn is affected by malnutrition of the mother and the consequent low birth weight of the baby and in some cases they get born with certain deformities because of the inadequate growth inputs supplied through the pregnant mother.

That the fear ignorant people carry, that the foetus will grow big and hurt safe delivery has been the main reason for depriving the pregnant woman of good and nourishing food. This practice of starving the pregnant and lactating mother continues and no scientific medical advice is heeded by the rural folk. If hopefully the woman is educated or well informed and has some rights there may be a change in her asserting to follow the best practices and avoid the rural unscientific superstitious apprehensions. From the very start, the unborn child suffers because of lack of empowerment of the mother.

Thus continues the saga of deprivation, discrimination distress and death leading to IMR and MMR. This threat to the very survival of both the infant and the mother remains uncontrolled even today. The visible and invisible pressures on the woman in the village have been explained in the text of this study and also through the empirical evidence collected during our investigations. They amply justify the contention that lack of empowerment of women due to socio-economic causes and determinants have been the main factors for the status of infant and maternal mortality as on today.

Whether one realizes the importance of the need for empowerment of women for reducing both infant and maternal mortality or not, the lack of empowerment is a stumbling block in maternal and child health and survival.

5

CONCLUSION AND RECOMMENDATIONS

In the previous sections of this report, we have highlighted what our research team, and, my State visitations, have revealed to us. We have tried to reproduce the same in an objective manner. We have found several direct and indirect measures undertaken by the official apparatus right down to the grass roots level in the country. Consider that India has in several states around 62,000 villages including its hamlets and remote settlements in the countryside and adding, to it, the remote areas and the coastal periphery. We also have people living in the mountainous areas at a higher altitude, and numerous tribal settlements all over India. Let us not ignore people living in Andaman Nicobar and Lakshwadeep group of islands. Thus India is a large human system with a cultural plurality characteristic of its people.

Against this backdrop and reality of India, can our Planners and Policy makers honestly say, "we have reached all of them with our plans and developmental recipies and programmes"? This report which covers only a few districts and a few villages, therefore, can at best be just indicative in nature.

We shall not go into the issue of governance here. But if the Ninth Five Year Plan's midterm appraisal Volume III is looked at, then this study's logic compels us to agree with the official review that, "In large number of policies and rules act against the interests of the poor. There is need for putting pro-poor policies in place". We further agree that the government needs to evolve a culture which help, promote, "the successful implementation of developmental programmes".

The question is, are the current delivery systems are in a position to optimally utilize funds and realise the goals fully with respect to IMR and MMR. The Experiential evidence, no matter of which official review, we examine, or look at our meager findings, they reconfirm that the Indian implementation of IMR and MMR reduction programmes are not substantial enough. Specially, if we look at the schemes relating to 'Primary Health, Primary Education, Watershed Development, Employment of local people and Women in particular. All these, notwithstanding the role of Panchayats can be crucial. A key question that stares in our face is if the Panchayatiraj mechanism is in any way helping in minimizing the tragedy associated with the IMR and MMR?

The problems are far too many, if the implementation aspects are looked at, be it responding to the needs of women or the issue of accountability for effective grassroot functionary's role including allied financial management, these do deserve to be made more effective. The question is how? People are people. In a country where malpractices thrive, can we say several ASHAs and a few invisible ANMs, can deliver "the direct welfare measure" and could salvage the local IMR/MMR tragedy? We need to look hard at the grass root functionaries versus needy people's large numbers. Besides, health care, do these people have any recourse to a responsive legal system at the grass root level? How can poor people invoke and seek assistance to any kind of justice system? After all infant killing is a heinous crime.

A word may be mentioned about administrative malpractice. An input that our field workers provided us from Andhra Pradesh was from Mehaboobnagar district; it said that an ANM - midwife was engaged in selling the new born babies on the side for a price anywhere between Rs. 5000 to Rs. 1,50,000. She would tell the poor mothers whom she delivered of, that the child was born dead. It is more than apparent that we have to stimulate and invigorate the Panchayatiraj system to ensure local vigilance, honest implementation of our Plan schemes as was stated categorically in *the foreword of Volume I of the Five Year Plan, 2002-2007, entitled, Dimensions and Strategies^ wherein it was said that, "Effective delivery of basic social services to our people cannot be ensured unless the institutions that are charged with these functions are made accountable to the people themselves. For this it is necessary to empower the PR institutions by transferring to them both functions and resources. The PRIs must become the cutting edge of our 3 tier political structure and the focal point of democratic decentralization".*

It would be insane and Churlish to suggest that the Planning Commission and the Policy making personnel are not trying to invigorate to the best of their effort for the most needy sector of Rural India. What is it then that the Government of India's plethora of schemes are missing? For the indirect steps, they are regulating ground water use, they are stepping up development by industrializing locally and also integrating agricultural markets. They have introduced the Kisan Credit Cards and allied reforms to strengthen the economic base for the poor people. Like this there are several *indirect attempts* which *inter-alia* may help the economic empowerment of our rural women as well.

However, when it comes to improving the quality of life, notwithstanding our schemes of financing health care. In the context of demographic picture of our nation, even when the 10th Plan, provided for and encouraged to provide certain health care services free of cost integral to the different aspects of National Family Welfare programmes, can we say it is enough or, that official indices concerning the health care infrastructure have been examined was in a satisfactory

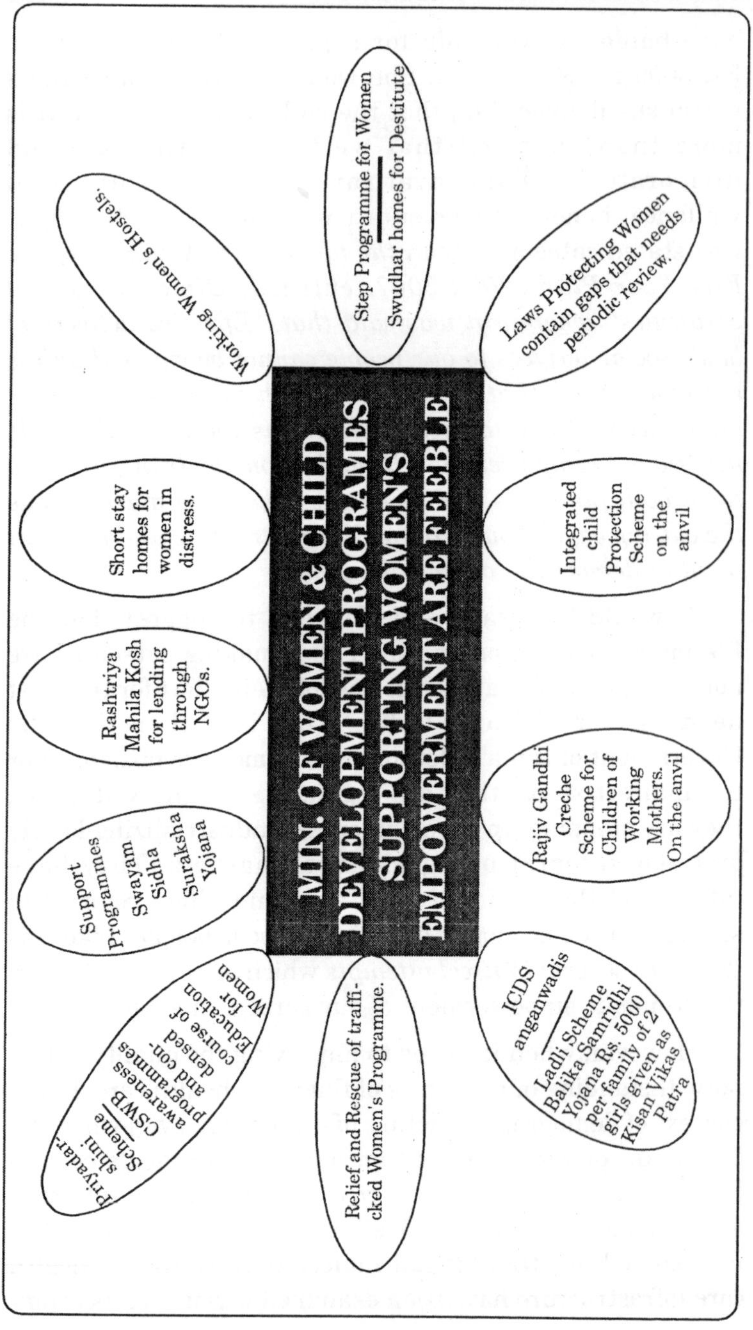
MIN. OF WOMEN & CHILD
DEVELOPMENT PROGRAMES
SUPPORTING WOMEN'S
EMPOWERMENT ARE FEEBLE
Step Programme for Women
Swudhar homes for Destitute
Working Women's Hostels.
Laws Protecting Women contain gaps that needs periodic review.
Short stay homes for women in distress.
Integrated child Protection Scheme on the anvil
Rashtriya Mahila Kosh for lending through NGOs.
Rajiv Gandhi Creche Scheme for Children of Working Mothers. On the anvil
Support Programmes Swayam Sidha Suraksha Yojana
ICDS anganwadis
Ladli Scheme Balika Samridhi Yojana Rs. 5000 per family of 2 girls given as Kisan Vikas Patra
Relief and Rescue of traffi-cked Women's Programme.
Priyadar-shini Scheme
CSWB awareness programmes and con-densed course of Education for Women

manner? A Plan review indicated that free welfare packet release and utilisation varied from district to district and from village to village; we too in our research noticed it. Of course, now a realization and a change is visible wherein an effort to reassess the health plan measures are being made to make district-specific health, nutrition and Family Planning needs.

However we need to face the crucial question, why a visible dichotomy and mismatch between good policies and the welfare of the needy specifically lingers on, when it is about IMR and MMR. Here, *one cannot help but say that in spite of all our plans and our schemes, they have proved ineffective in coping with the stranglehold of traditions, taboos, personalized beliefs, caste considerations and religious constraints. Because these limitations and numerous societal cultural handicaps inbuilt in the life of the people, do escape the benefits of economic development.* Can we say our Plan provisions have taken all the local factors into account? Do these social indices articulate each Plan's technical notes? Further more, are our national targets in place? If not, then what is the missing factor, one or too many?

The above question arise because grassroots impact is in no way uplifting enough to curb IMR/MMR. Our policies have not quite alter our people-mind sets? If this does not happen, then, our best efforts and programmes and strategies for equity and social justice, will fail to transform our society. Consequently, IMR and MMR will continue, even if it be at a reduced scale.

As referred to in the earlier sections also, this report only addresses two key factors. Firstly, we are asking, can we think of new direct and indirect innovative schemes to reduce IMR and MMR. This may help our Planners and Policy makers to fine tune their existing schemes and programmes which are praiseworthy but are not helping much (with great humility I must also say that in none of the State villages visited by us- they had any idea what

Planning Commission is all about).

The second question that we are addressing here is based on our firm belief that we need to do whatever we can and as much as we can, in as many ways in which we can, *we better empower the woman.* If this happens and when it happens, we are confident that an empowered woman will become the most powerful auxiliary and support measure to reduce IMR and MMR.

Direct and Indirect Plan Schemes, Deserve Fresh Look and New Emphasis

We now turn to some ideas of the direct and indirect schemes which can help us in our mission of getting rid of this social malaise and scourge of infant and maternal mortality. One small point we would like to repeatedly emphasise is, that the policy makers should continue to remember is, that the Indian populace lives, simultaneously, in several centuries time frame and concomitant practices. As hinted earlier, therefore, some Plan schemes, all, propounded by the First Five Year Plan and by successive thinkers may still be valid in some parts of India. However, that does not prevent us from fresh creative thinking for and towards future.

What we found during our research in the villages of six states is that the villagers are not aware of what the National Rural Health Mission stands for, and what exactly do the health policies, offer to the poor rural folk. Out of curiosity the villagers have gone and seen the Anganwadis, the primary health centre and the sub-health centre in the village. These village level workers shared with us their woes that it has been very difficult for them to convince the village women to believe that these centres are opened in the village only for their benefit. Is it a case of credibility deficit?

The ANMs and Anganwadi workers narrated to our research team that it took more than a year and a half to make them agree to go for the immunization and vaccination of children and pregnant mothers, particularly in Rajasthan and Andhra Pradesh. The women, though refused these procedures for themselves but agreed to have them for their children.

For people who are deeply rooted in superstition, and cultural practices that are inimical to the modern medi-care, it has been a yeoman task for the village level Anganwadi workers and the health workers to win village women's faith and confidence. Currently people are attracted to the *nashta* (snacks) given by the Anganwadis to the children and pregnant and lactating mothers. Our team found that the maize balls given as *nashta* to children and women are neither tasty nor filling. When we told the workers that in Southern Indian states, cooked nashta is given to children and women, they said they would also be doing the same in a few months. It is the poor families who were visiting the centres and not the upper caste women. (The most caste minded area in Haryana is NUH, where even the Muslims practise caste system. For them, the Centres, are of no use).

Health Service Delivery System and Allied Infrastructural Issues

Talking to village women, our team could realize how entrenched a life they are living, still caught in the age old customs and beliefs, and, in evil spirits and taboos, imposed by their communities generation after generation. In the 21 century their world exists in the shadow of the 2nd century. *In this existence the women have also no freedom of choice, no decision making power or of movement without permission of their husbands and in-laws. In such a situation, unless the health service delivery reaches to their doorstep it would be ineffective; it is not easy for the local women to avail of these services though specifically meant for them, because of the many restrictions that they face day after day.*

Let us now turn to a few inadequacies in the delivery system. We found that the health service delivery is through the primary health centre and that the number of staff appointed are not adequate to cater fully to the village collective needs. The key person in the PHC is the ANM who visits each village once a month. The doctor visits once in three months, that too for an hour and a half. The multipurpose male worker who is to dispense medicines is often found absent, or, he is out on a visit to the village households for collecting population related records. While the PHCs profess to provide 24 hours service for cases of delivery and for family planning procedures, the inadequacy of staff is one reason for villagers refusal to depend on their services, apart from the problem of commuting distances locally. For them, an untrained, unskilled, local dai (midwife) remains still an, "angel of mercy", Is she really?

Besides, Haryana and in other States visited by us, we also found that the dual appointment of both permanent and contract ANMs had created confusion in the minds of the village women. The policy of employing ANMs on contract, on retirement of the permanent ones, is not encouraging women to opt for the new ANMs services. They would prefer to revert back to their traditional dais in whom they have enough faith. Other reason is that being a contract employee, the new ANM may not stay in the village and may also attend to private delivery cases outside the assigned village. The ANMs are not easily available. Hence it is this recruitment policy that needs change, because it is not matching with the requirements of the village women's needs and that of their children. Our team also found in the villages of Haryana, in Harchandpur and Rethoj, small children were having chest cold and there was neither a doctor nor even an ANM to attend to the children. When one of our team members told the women to apply 'ajwain oil', to the chest if nothing else is available, the women replied that 'bhoot' (ghost) will stick to the chest if, "ajwain" is used'. It may appear irrational to the urbanites, but the key question is how to change such an old mind-set?

As far as ASHAs go, it is true that engaging ASHAs as

announced by the government, one for every village, is a welcome step. Yet in the places, visited by us, we could find only one ASHA in more than 10 PHC areas. In Maharashtra in the Nashik district, they have not yet thought of engaging ASHAs, and in other states, we were informed that they will soon be appointed. The least said about Uttarakhand would be better.

The point that is being made here is that even if the State is extending its health related assistance to the recipient *i.e*: expectant mothers, the State machinery has almost failed to establish a credible relationship. Surely we can sympathise with the village health care workers who, sometimes, have long distances and difficult terrains to negotiate. It is typical of the State of Uttarakhand. Even in other places, we need to remedy a situation in hospitals where, doctors are seldom present and are on leave. Medicines in-variably are just not available. On the one hand the supply side infrastructure for health care is awaiting for the needy to arrive; on the other hand the demand side "needy" does not feel motivated enough to seek external assistance, and would rather depend on the known, and available traditional local dais. Even if when the village women do muster courage, often they do not receive the required assistance, either from the PHC or, the ANM or the ASHA. Therefore, our Policy makers should take due remedial attention to the aforesaid all-pervasive phenomena in the Indian villages and several different remote areas. Of course, the key question would remain on, "How to convince their women folk?" If this is done, it may contribute towards some reduction in IMR and MMR. (As a contrast let us remember that even AIIMS, where 1000s of doctors are catering to more than 5000 patients each day. Here we have only an ANM and an ASHA. The economically empowered villagers who are to commute distances to come to AIIMS. In fact they form 50% of thousands of patients, visiting big urban hospitals. .... contrast it to the pathetic ratio of one ANM or an ASHA for 5000 plus population of a single village and consider what may become of staff who may often serve a Block that may have more than 100 villages seeking health care.

Role of Anganwadi Workers and ANM's

We need to look at two additional points here. As they also deserve scrutiny and remedial measures to augment the role of Anganwadis and ANMs.

The Anganwadi workers along with ANMs are expected to attend to women for antenatal care and post natal care; care of infants and provide for women and children for immunization and vaccination needs. The Anganwadi workers also counsel them on the advantages of these procedures and about the nutrient requirements, during pregnancy.

Our team, however, found that in all the Six States, the presence of children in the Anganwadis was sporadic. In some villages they were 10 or 11 kids but in other villages they even numbered 80 plus children. All the children were coming for the *'nashta'* only. They were seldom engaged by the Anganwadi workers in teaching them good sanitary practices, even through, " Role Play". It is apparent that for this, we need to have highly trained Anganwadi workers. The ANM's have hardly any time for such activities.

Our researchers also got the impression that the majority of women of the villages strongly felt that the ANMs are only occasional visitors. Hence they cannot entirely depend on them as ANMs are not available daily and certainly not during emergencies.

We need to extend our sympathies to the above mentioned healthcare workers for more than one reason. By virtue of their duties assigned to them and by their qualifications the Anganwadi workers and ASHAs for all intents and purposes, are not necessarily health workers. Their role is limited to act as either counsellors or as conduits between the pregnant woman in need and the PHCs or hospitals. The question does arise, if we can enhance the number of health-oriented ANMs and compensate them financially to stay in the village. We can then achieve ANM's better interface with village women? The real remedy thus lies not only in doubling up of their numbers, but also of the status of their training and skills? At the moment, it is not only minimal, if not sub-standard, for them to qualify as the local health MESSIAH to reduce IMR and MMR.

We, therefore, strongly recommend the following: Apart from increasing the strength of the ANMs, it is important to upgrade their female health related and allied knowledge level. Their presence in the village will enhance better assistance to village women. They will inspire more faith in modern medicine as against the village womens faith in the local customary practices. Their frequent visits to the local tantrics, sadhus, priests and peers may thus gradually stop. If the ANMs are convincing enough, the village women will not throw away as it happens today the iron and folic acid tablets offered as part of the nutrition programme.

We sincerely believe that the role of Panchayats would be the most significant input and turning point to reduce IMR and MMR. Every Panchayat firstly appoints a Health Committee. If these committees begin to work with creative zeal and compassion and take conducive steps towards reducing IMR & MMR, we will not only be achieving our goal of due reduction of IMR and MMR but we will also set up a yardstick to assess the effectiveness of the Panchayati Raj system.

We feel emboldened to recommend this because in many States visited by us, we did not come across a single Health Committee that has been set up by the local Panchayats. We think that all States should ensure it post-haste.

Other ideas: When we begin to search creative, direct or indirect remedial measures to reduce IMR and MMR we do realize that IMR and MMR is shrouded by numerous causes and determinants personal and local to a given settlement. There is no one single remedy that can be attempted to reduce the deleterious effects of these beliefs. But numerous support systems can be thought of besides, the Public Health System, *THE SELF HELP GROUPS*, and voluntary NGOs support need to be activated. The most important of all tasks is how to influence grass roots customary social behaviour and gently influence, atleast, the leaders of the local community and castes towards elementary modernity. Hopefully they may further in turn motivate the rural folk.

STEPPING UP OF TRAINING AND MASS AWARENESS PROGRAMMES

The Government's plan to train PHC staff as multi-purpose health workers in curative skills is a welcome step. But what is ailing PHCs is lack of supplies and medicine, even for the qualified doctors, to dispense. There is an urgent need to equip near empty PHCs with medicines and other needed resources by way of staff, equipment to make them effective medi-care service providers. Equally important is the intensive training of the PHC staff to develop a more adequate health care delivery system. Even modern doctors need to be trained to make them more sensitive to the villager's needs. These doctors need to think of themselves as 'authority' figure. This will enable them to pass on valuable health ideas to villagers in a manner the villagers can understand. Hopefully it may add to the villagers quality of life. Besides such sensitivity may have indirect and direct impact towards the reduction of IMR and MMR. Responsive health planning and medical orientation will require the benefit of anthropological research into regional health profile. This will help planners to assess their right manpower, and supplies. If training gets supplemented by the region specific modules, then we can impart a new knowledge.

And above all it is necessary to equip all Rural Medical Practitioners (RMPs) and to be given better knowledge of allopathic medicines. They can become helpful change agents in the village, since villagers have faith in them.

NGO'S CAN BE ADDITIONAL TRAINERS

To some extent the health culture of a community gets reflected in the health behaviour of the rural people. The introduction of the rural health delivery system by the government, can be effective only *if the villager's cultural perception accept, and sees the public health care interventions, as purposive and useful.* We could encourage NGOs, assisted by the State, to help orient husbands and mothers-in-law to become more caring a person towards the expectant mothers and the girl child.

In a feedback from Rajasthan, our research group was informed how a local NGO introduced the 'Role Play' approach. It was made a tool to train a group of husbands to sensitise them towards expectant mothers. These husbands were asked to dress like a woman, pillows were tied to their tummy to make them feel that they were heavy like the pregnant women. They were asked to cook with 3-4 children wailing around them. Simultaneously, they were to take care of the children while they were cooking. Besides their heads were totally covered, their face not visible and they faced smoking chulhas, too. Finally, they were asked, "will you agree to live like this for nine months? In just one hour it was reported that this short experience did make some impact on the participating husbands and their perception of woman did alter a wee - bit. Similar programmes can be designed for mothers-in-law, to not consider a girl, "a parayadhan" and an expensive commodity or only a machine to produce 'boy' child.

A doctor in the group explained later, how a pregnant woman should be treated; why there is an urge to kill a girl child when the woman has gone through the same pain and suffering as she would have gone through by delivering a male child." *The truth of the matter is, and it is very significant that, invariably, the killer of the girl child, in majority of the cases, is the mother-in-law who demands of the dais to kill the newborn baby girl.*

It is now common knowledge that in the State of Rajasthan in Badmer district a single marriage took place after a period of 110 years. Here there are villages after villages, in the same region, where bachelors live who are aged 65 and 75 years old. In fact the dowry is given by the bridegroom to get a bride. But alas, there are no marriageable girls available.

They have long back been put to death and the practice of infanticide persists. In the State of Tamil Nadu, however, infanticide was prevalent and for long it still continues in some hilly pockets. The law and the policy of the Government, however has failed to fully stop incidence of infanticide. But innovative approach of *"Cradle Baby Scheme"* has certainly saved hundreds of girl infants.

THE 'PALNA' OR CRADLE BABY SCHEME. OUR PRIME RECOMMENDATION TO THE CENTRAL AND STATE GOVERNMENT

When incidents of female infanticide in some remote villages in Madurai and Salem districts were brought to the notice of the Government, by the media, responding immediately, the Government of Tamil Nadu started a reception centre at *Usilampatti in Madurai District.* It was run by the Indian Council for Child Welfare with the help of government funds during early 1990's. The services offered in Usilampatti were:

(i) Running reception centres to receive unwanted babies.

(ii) Counselling of pregnant mothers and their families.

(iii) Support services - education, training and creating need based opportunities for livelihood for women.

(iv) Sponsorship Programmes.

(v) Hostel facilities to complete schooling.

(vi) Local Day-care centre for working mothers.

During 1992 when such awareness creation was on in Madurai-incidents of female infanticide in remote rural areas of Salem district too were reported in the media.

To counter their menace of female infanticide in certain parts of Tamil Nadu "Cradle Baby Scheme." Was first implemented, from 1992, in the Salem District. Under this scheme cradles were placed in important places such as the Government hospitals, Primary Health Centres, Collectorates / District Social Welfare Offices to enable the parents to drop their female babies if they are unable to bring them up so that the Government may take care of such babies. As per G.O. (D) No. 11, Social Welfare and NMP Department dated 23.03.1993 it was stated that the Government have taken steps to curtail female infanticide and all the Primary Health Centres and Anganwadi Centres were instructed to place cradles in Salem District to rescue the girl babies from being killed. Later on the Government in G.O. Ms. No.88, Social Welfare and NMP Department dated 30.03.93 issued an order to set up cradles in Salem District near the Primary Health Centres and in vulnerable areas of Salem District so as to facilitate the mothers to leave their unwanted babies in the cradles.

This was considered a measure to rescue the girl babies from the jaws of death. In the G.O. cited, the Director of Social Welfare, has been instructed to formulate and implement the programme and for creating awareness among the people. In the same G.O. it has been stated that "the children received, may be given in adoption" and it was instructed that, "the Director of Social Defence and the District Collector, Salem shall make efforts to encourage adoption". The children who could not be given in adoption were advised, to be handed over to reputed Non-

Governmental Organisations".

It is interesting to note how, in the mean time, the Consulate General of Japan came forward to fund the programme to a tune of Rs.22,40,440 during March 1995. A building was constructed at the cost of Rs.5.50 lakh and a jeep, an Ambulance and an Audiovisual van were purchased for bringing the children, educating the mass and propagating against the evils of female infanticide.

From the year 1992 to 5/2001 the Salem Cradle Baby Home has received 150 children as detailed below:

		Male	*Female*	*Total*
	No. of children received	0	150	150
1.	Children died to disease	0	40	40
2.	Returned to parents	0	14	14
3.	School going children in orphanage	0	23	23
4.	In country adoption	0	39	39
5.	Inter country adoption	0	28	28

From the year 2001 onwards the Government in G.O. Ms. No. 158 Social Welfare and NMP Department dated 24.10.2001 it was decided to "revitalise the cradle baby scheme", and accordingly, reception centres, were started in Madurai, Theni, Dindigul and Dharmapuri. As per the Government instructions 188 cradles were placed in all the Primary Health Centres / Office of the District Social Welfare Officers in districts of Madurai, Theni, Dindigul, Dharmapuri, Namakkal and Erode..Further the Tamil Nadu Government also sanctioned a sum of Rs.12.96 lakhs for the starting of reception Centres in Madurai, Theni, Dindigul and Dharmapuri. The main function of the Reception centres was to receive the babies, to provide shelter, "Medical facilities and hand them over to the adoption agency". The Government provided funds for the maintenance of reception centres on an annual basis.

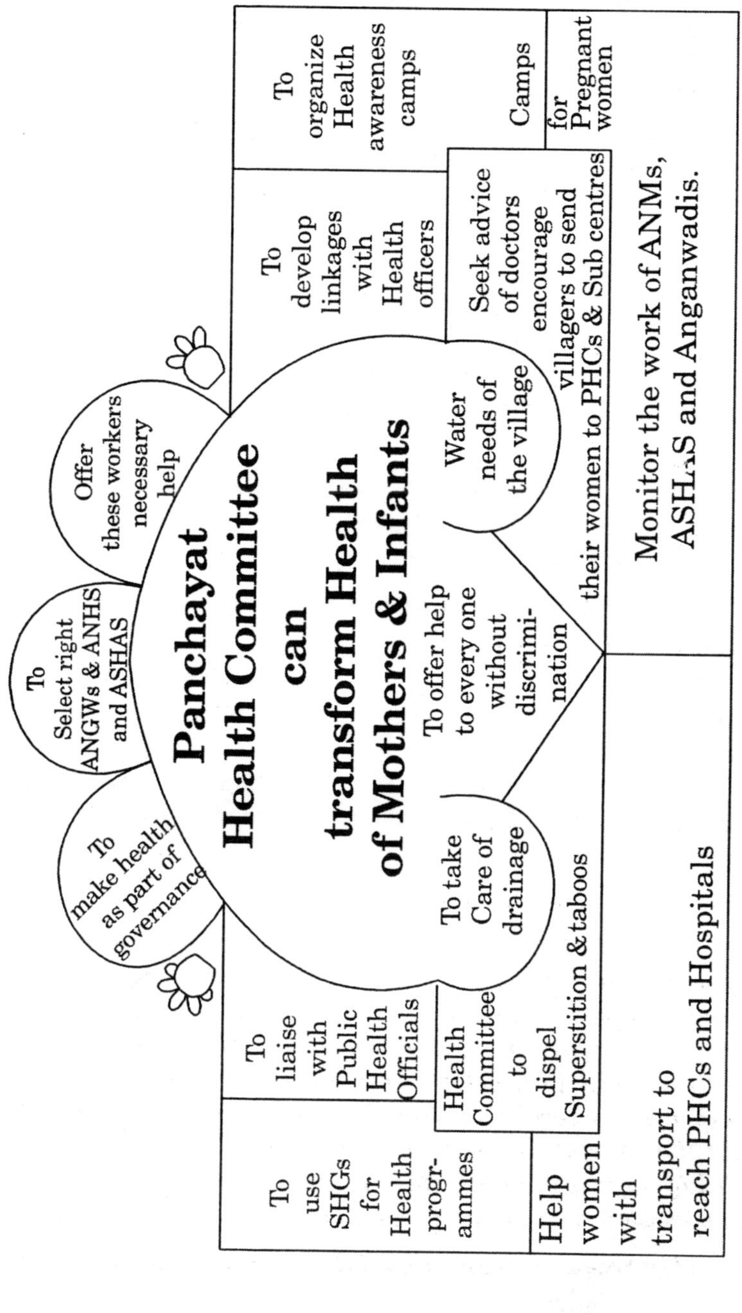
Panchayat Health Committee can transform Health of Mothers & Infants
To make health as part of governance
To Select right ANGWs & ANHS and ASHAS
Offer these workers necessary help
To develop linkages with Health officers
To organize Health awareness camps
Camps
for Pregnant women
Seek advice of doctors encourage villagers to send their women to PHCs & Sub centres
Monitor the work of ANMs, ASHAS and Anganwadis.
Water needs of the village
To offer help to every one without discrimi- nation
To take Care of drainage
To liaise with Public Health Officials
Health Committee to dispel Superstition & taboos
To use SHGs for Health progr- ammes
Help women with transport to reach PHCs and Hospitals

At all the reception centres in Tamil Nadu, they are having pucca infrastructure facilities along with life saving drugs, life saving equipment, telephone, water and electricity facilities and with adequate staff. Funds are also provided for the purchase of medicine, clothing, feeding and for other contingencies. Apart from these 5 reception centres, cradles have also been placed at the Collectorates and District Social Welfare Offices. They have been officially designated as "cradle" points.

As envisaged in G.O. No. 88 SW & NMP Dept., dt. 30.03.93, the children received in the reception centres were handed over to 21 licensed adoption agencies (both in and inter country) for rehabilitation through adoption programme.

This 'Palna' called the 'Cradle Baby Scheme' can easily be replicated in all States. This is one of the visible and direct ways to protect the new born infant from death.

Some Additional Thoughts on State-Local Health Related Inter-Face

We strongly feel that a responsive health planning and medical orientation will require deep anthropological research into regional health sectors, whch will help planners to fine tune the current schemes to grassroot, variable realities, from village to village, district to district and state to state.

Our Recommendation

Since the PHCs play a pivotal role in the Government sponsored Rural Health Service System and as the empirical surveys reveal that they are in disarray and do deserve hightened training and orientation. There is adequate political will to develop rural health services. We should respond to several public health workers who have pointed out that in spite of their concern for the village women and children's health needs, there is still a lack of co-ordination and commitment of the official apparatus at the village level.

Our research team also felt that the Panchayats. the

PHCs, ICDS, Health workers all work in isolation. There is considerable degree of unmet needs for maternal and child health services. There is no collaborative and co-ordinated functioning of these agencies and other institutions. Therefore the efforts have not helped in reduction of IMR and MMR.

Besides this, it is recommended that the recruitment of staff to the Anganwadis, primary health centres and ASHAs to the PHCs, Sub-Centres need a thorough review. ANMs regular home visits to counsel women on maternal and child health care has to be regular and has to be constantly monitored

Some Legal Points Concerning IMR and MMR

1. The practice of foeticide, the killing of the unborn child and later committing infanticide are cognizable offences. They are non-bailable too.
2. Solemnising of child marriages is against the law prohibiting child marriage. Marriage of girls below the age of 18 years is also prohibited.
3. Dowry giving and taking are offences under the dowry prohibition act.
4. The prenatal diagnostic techniques tests with a view to reveal the sex of the foetus is banned by law.
5. Only the Medical Termination of Pregnancy Act enables women to terminate pregnancies for certain valid reasons.The MTP Act empowers accredited hospitals and doctors to undertake such operations.
6. Domestic violence perpetrated on women is prohibited by law so also is the torturing and abuse of children and women.
7. Registration of births, marriages and deaths have been initiated by states not merely for purposes of census records but to ensure a variety of safety measures to the infant/child, and the mother.

The lack of awareness of our laws is a negative feature. The national health and other policies on empowerment of women, alas, receive a scant or no attention from the rural community. Abetment to such offences are also cognizable and severely punishable; yet it continues, in our large country. This was also confirmed by our field investigators. In the villages visited by them, none of these laws or policies, have been followed or obeyed by the local village community. One can attribute ignorance for such inaction, yet one cannot ignore the fact that the social disregard to the laws appear more powerful than the laws themselves. *This dishonouring of the law is again the outcome of strong socio-economic causes and the cultural way of life and lack of awareness. Such a situation is not at all conducive to reducing infant and maternal mortality rates.*

One can deduce from such a village scenario which is bereft of the respect of law besides, being indifferent to the modern medical care. What hope then can we have in preventing the rising/stagnating IMR and MMR. This state of affair does seem very bleak. *It calls for innovative programmes and strategies towards multi-pronged attempt to change the behaviour of the villagers.*

WOMEN'S EMPOWERMENT: A SURE RECIPE TO REDUCE IMR AND MMR

(A) Healthcare empowerment: needs massive awareness and contact strategy.

1. Available health infrastructure specially in rural areas is too inadequate to cater to women who are half of the existing population.
2. *The Indian planning being predominantly an economic process, offers a mis-match to respond to our tradition-bound superstitious rural ethos. This public policy is not able to break this superstitious life cycle handed over from one generation to another.*

Right to life and her safety and of her children.	Right to question superstition and harmful practices.	Right to utilise governmental facilities created for Women and the girl child	Right to increase Woman's age at marriage.	Right to conceive at a mature age for safe motherhood.
Right to nutrition during pregnancy and after delivery.	Right to decide the size of her family.	Right to sanitation and hygiene and good environment	Right to decision making on matters concerning her person and family.	Right to childcare as per medical advice specially of the girl child.

POLICIES FOCUSSED ON WOMEN'S EMPOWERMENT NEED TO BE STEPPED UP TO ENSURE HER NUMEROUS RIGHT

Right to breast feed her baby.	Right of the girl child to pursue studies in Primary and High school	Right to cross the old patriarchical values and of women's subordination.	Right to resist violence and right to seek community support.	Right to seek medi-care services and intervention before and after delivery.
Right to employment outside home and contribute to better child care	Right to economic stability and sustainability.	Right to equal resources and equal attention by members of the family.	Right of mobility and freedom to communicate with Parents and Friends.	Right to be aware of laws and invoke laws in her favour.

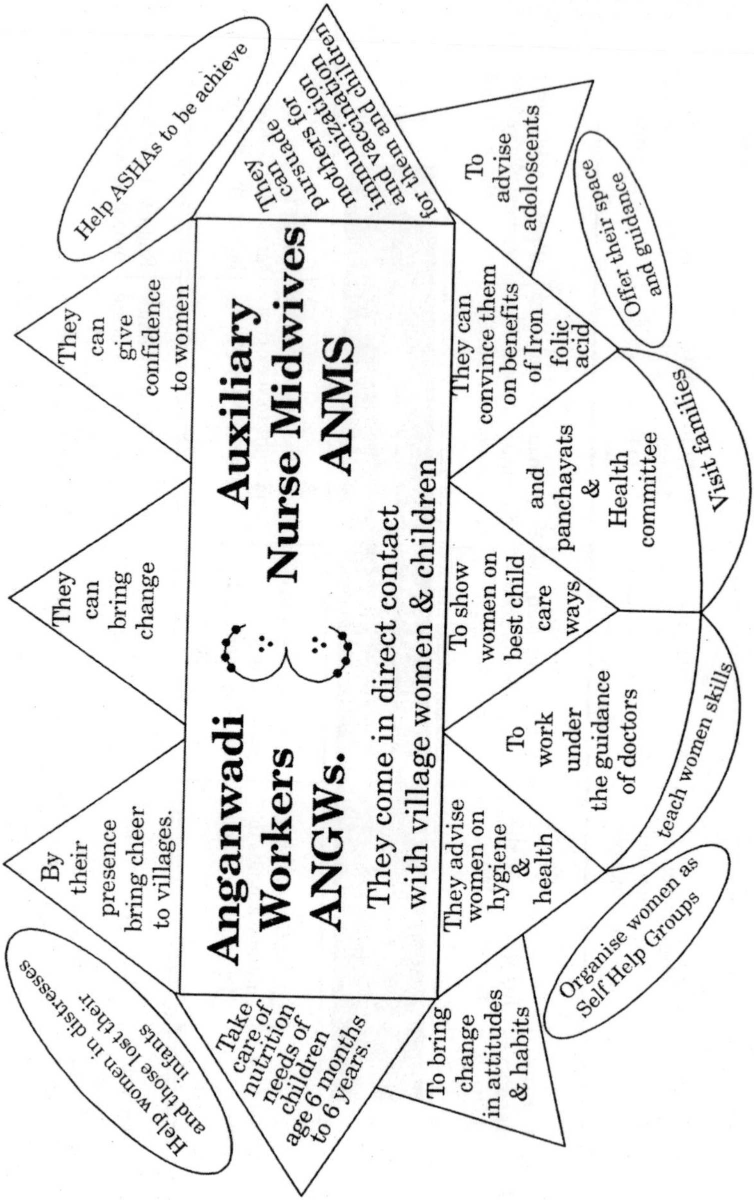
Anganwadi Workers ANGWs.
&
Auxiliary Nurse Midwives ANMS
They come in direct contact with village women & children
By their presence bring cheer to villages.
They can bring change
They can give confidence to women
Help ASHAs to be achieve
They can persuade mothers for immunization and vaccination for them and children
To advise adoloscents
Offer their space and guidance
They can convince them on benefits of Iron folic acid
and panchayats & Health committee
Visit families
To show women on best child care ways
To work under the guidance of doctors
teach women skills
They advise women on hygiene & health
Organise women as Self Help Groups
To bring change in attitudes & habits
Take care of nutrition needs of children age 6 months to 6 years.
Help women in distresses and those lost their infants

3. *Behaviour modification is a big communication challenge to grapple with and there is need to retune the planning process for the social sector.*
4. Identification and removing of a plethora of handicaps suffered by women including lack of autonomy in decision making even about her own health and that of her infant are imperative and important.
5. We, therefore, need to step-up ten times massive awareness programmes for the rural folk to make them grasp positive information about health to their own advantage.

(B) A triple insurance scheme for women's empowerment: We need to introduce a triple insurance scheme ensuring *Health, Education and Employment* for all women specially for those living below poverty line.

(C) Offer nutritious and cooked meals to children of anganwadis and pregnant and lactating mothers.

Women's empowerment in the household and community, needs integrated planning with multisectoral policy assuring economic cover and opportunities for free health, education, right to life and survival and freedom of choice and right to regular employment and income. **Unless the woman is liberated and enabled to seek health care, any amount of superstructure with adequate infrastructural facilities will be futile. Empowering women to take their own decisions and to free them from the patriarchical hold is a top priority for Planners and Policy makers.**

For a Successful Health Service Delivery

From our study, it is our finding, that it is necessary to ensure greater synergy between ICDS and the Health system to fully involve Anganwadi workers in maternal, neonatal and postneonatal care at the household and communuity levels in the rural areas.

- Develop sustainable models of obstetric-neonatal services at PHCs, CHCs and district hospitals.
- Renewed efforts are needed to finish the unfinished agenda of routine immunization and ORT. We need to scale up community skilled birth attendants scheme to meet the long standing need of providing skilled birth attendants in the community. Involve Panchayati Raj institutions (PRIs) in saving infants, neonats and post-neonats.
- There is need to prepare advocacy and educational materials targeted to Panchayati Raj leaders at district,sub-district and village levels.
- Demonstrate sustainable models of public-private partnership for survival of infants.
- Establish a partnership of all concerned NGOs, ANMs, AWWs, SHGs in reducing IMR by involving them to serve as a platform for advocacy, strategic deliberations, programme support and experience learning.

EDUCATION : AWARENESS AND PEOPLE'S EMPOWERMENT

The social, cultural and health conditions related to low status of women in India have a negative impact on child survival; improvements in female education, nutrition and the use of maternal health care services would help in reducing infant mortality.

- Girls have higher mortality rate than boys from the age one month to 5 years and receive less health care. Eliminating gender difference in mortality rates would help reduce child and infant mortality rates.
- India needs to reassess the country's child mortality

reduction goals and go forward with enhanced integrated approach for child health and nutrition.

- Considering the difference in infant and child mortality performance between states, stratified child health policies are needed to take into account, state specified epidemiological and demographic patterns and key determinants.

NEEDED STRATEGIES

- Identification of high risk blocks showing high infant deaths especially female infanticide.
- Establish Health Co-ordination Committees involving Panchayat leaders, ward members, medical officers and health staff, revenue department officials, voluntary agencies, community leaders and other influencial persons at village/block and district levels.
- Functions of this committee would be to (i) identify families with more than one female child.
- Encourage these to avail all health services for safe pregnancy, delivery and child survival and curbing infanticide practices.
- Highlighting government schemes for the benefit of women and girl child.
- To involving adolescent girls groups and PRI groups for health issues related to body mapping, reproductive health, family welfare, girl child protection, institutional delivery, to eliminate sex determination tests and work for gender equality.
- To introduce the cradle baby scheme of Tamil Nadu to prevent babies from infanticide.
- To establish operation theatres in PHCs to facilitate family planning services and medical termination of pregnancies.
- To ensure early registration of pregnancies, and for

early detection of high risk cases, improving institutional deliveries, providing skill development training to health staff on new born resuscitation techniques are important.

- To provide RCH training to medical staff, providing health management information system and also training for record management etc.
- To educate the mother of the merits of antenatal care, institutional delivery, importance of exclusive breast feeding, immunization, home care for diarrhoea; all these are meant to create awareness among family members to provide support to women during pregnancies and deliveries.
- *Revive the concept of delivery huts / waiting rooms for expectant mothers. Unifem earlier offered assistance to Haryana government and initiated this idea to start with in the State of Haryana; but this was for reasons not known have been discontinued. The delivery hut concept is innovative and at the same time of immense need for expectant mothers. This has to be revived if true efforts are on the anvil to reduce infant and maternal mortality.*

The Final Word

In so far as a set of recommendations go we have already catalogued the key ideas. One can multiply them by several hundreds. What can in reality get achieved is a separate matter. To give just one example the researchers of the study observed that "Sarva Siksha Abhiyan" has impact on education of children and specially girls. Our team feels that a **"Sarva Swasthya Abhiyan"** if started may step up the efforts to reduce IMR and MMR. This though deserves serious support, our implementation of Sarva Siksha Abhiyan, still is not upto national expectations.

Since there are no absolute answers for a total elimination of IMR and MMR, the ideal solution is that, we fine tune our direct and indirect interventions as reflected in our Five Year Plans and conferred policies that are being implemented by the Central Ministries and State Government, Administrative apparatus; and to reflect on the modus operandi to identify new ways and means, we need to reflect on the possible answers to an assorted set of questions given below:-

1. Is development an answer or a recipe for reduction of IMR and MMR?
2. Can stricter implementation of laws reduce IMR and MMR?
3. Can change in educational delivery at people's doorstep will help :
   (a) through public communication system?
   (b) audio-visual presentation?
   (c) through NGO's developing person to person contact for health?
4. Can incentives to poor families by way of :-
   (a) mid-day meals
   (b) food subsidy
   (c) subsidised shelter
   (d) free nutrition packets will help reduction of IMR and MMR?
5. Can employment to man and woman in the family help with support services like creche at work place, offered free or on nominal charges?
6. Is not empowerment of the woman, the answer?
7. Can massive training with free board and lodge followed by some economic activity like the SHGs - help the situation?
8. Reinforced tripartite enforcement structure at the village level for health service delivery - won't it help? With intensive training for Panchayats, ICDS personnel (the anganwadi workers), health

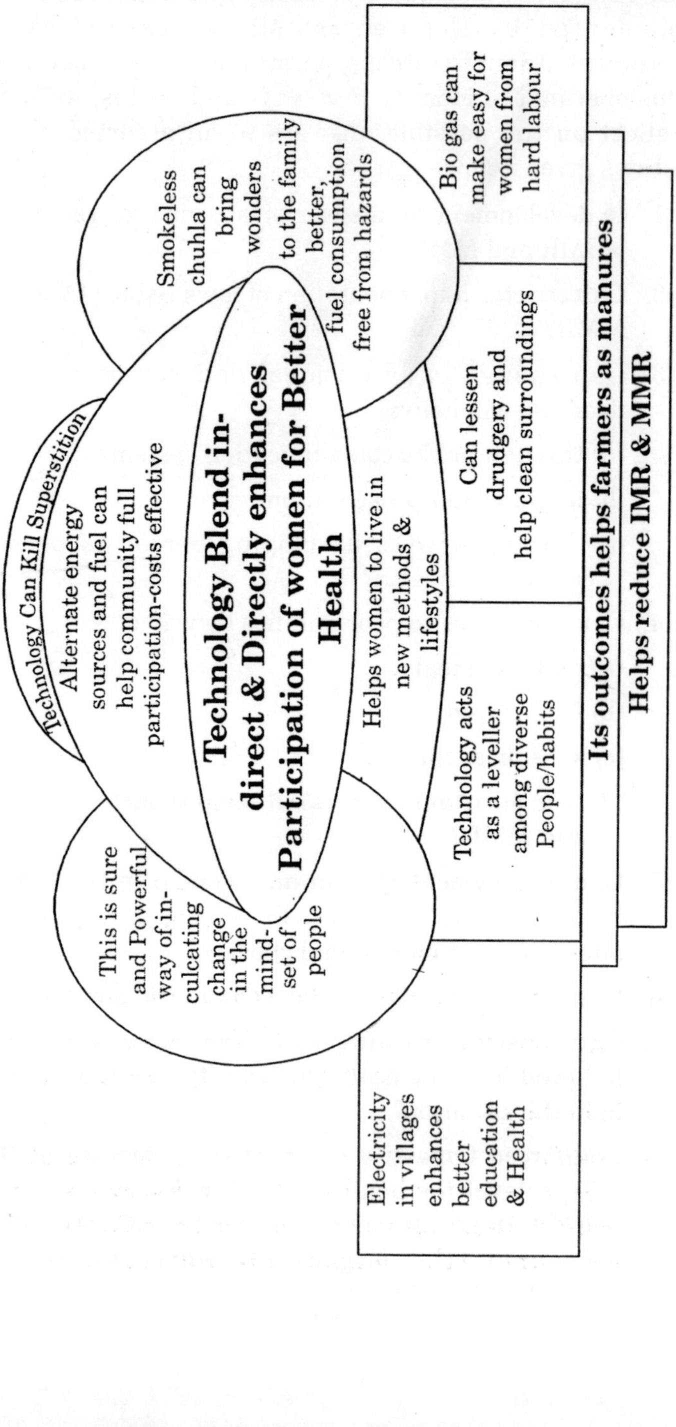
Technology Blend in-direct & Directly enhances Participation of women for Better Health
Technology Can Kill Superstition
Alternate energy sources and fuel can help community full participation-costs effective
Smokeless chuhla can bring wonders to the family better, fuel consumption free from hazards
This is sure and Powerful way of in-culcating change in the mind-set of people
Helps women to live in new methods & lifestyles
Bio gas can make easy for women from hard labour
Can lessen drudgery and help clean surroundings
Technology acts as a leveller among diverse People/habits
Electricity in villages enhances better education & Health
Its outcomes helps farmers as manures
Helps reduce IMR & MMR

personnel (of PHCs, ANMs and ASHAs).

9. Can we not have a village campaign:-
   (a) for Palna scheme
   (b) our village Swasthya campaign
   (c) SHGs for monitoring compulsory education of children specially the girls
   (d) for delivery huts
10. Can planning be?
    (a) women-centric
    (b) village-centric
    (c) development in a project mode
    (d) compulsory training for doctors in rural camps.
11. Can't we engage Local Committees:-
    (a) for health watch
    (b) education watch
    (c) foods security and distribution watch
    (d) public health watch

    all these to be made accountable to the tripartite village structure/committee.
12. Can we float awards for best performing village/ villagers.

The Stark and Frantally Staring Truth lies in the Question

Are our policies creating enough opportunities for transition of our people, when really they can create an appropriate modicum of transition, to freely move from one state of cultural web to a more emancipated environment, where *"dos and don'ts"* can be less painful and modern ways, more acceptable. Therefore this question persists as to what are those additional new innovative, creative ways and means which can accelerate the acceptance of scientific temper as against the *vice-like-grip* of superstition and people begin to live in an environment which can promote scientific healing for ills and allied health ailments pertaining to female sexuality and biology. This may, we believe, can help in the gradual reduction of IMR and MMR in India.

A search for new Policy, demands the active existence of an accelerated transition process, be it for housing, occupation, technology, health care, education, and massive awareness for maternal and child welfare and survival. a multi-sectoral, legal, health science and rationality approach is necessary.

We believe that the identification of new Plan schemes and programmes should have an organic character and forward movement. Once a system is installed, it should replicate itself. It should be sufficient and growing and with an evolutionary modicum. Of course, it has to be sustained by due fiscal support.

A nationwide support for technique and updated technology is a must. The important thing is that the real process of transition to be focussed for people's accepting modernity notwithstanding the historical grip of customs, traditions and caste compulsions. It should lead people forward, for an ongoing quest of our people, for fearless acceptance of current know how. A storehouse of awareness and knowledge, is out there awaiting the attention of our people. Let new science, new technology and new management be hereafter our guide. Ones this transition takes place India will surely be rid of IMR/MMR.

ANNEXURES

1. Empirical record sample
2. Questionnaire
3. Household facility survey
4. Parliament discussion on IMR
5. IMR/MMR ratio
6. SRS Bulletin

This annexure records quasi-empirical and quasioral history sampling (as recorded on the spot. In the villages visited) hardly 8 or 10 gave articulate response say out of 40 women.

In so far as Tamil Nadu is concerned, its official actions and policies are so positive that we have liberally recommended about the same in the main report.

(Maharashtra)	*Population : 2427 Male-1261—Female : 1166 Date 30-1-07*		
Rasegaon (Nasik)	*Sub-centre*	*Scheduled Tribe village*	*Articulate women deposed*
ANG Worker. Pushpa Sanjay Dhumane. Chandrakala-Supervisor ICDS-27 ANGWs. Shashikala-Asst. Child Dev. Proj. Officer 63 Children 3-6-yrs. 10 Children 0-3 yrs. 8 children 6 months-1 yr. While Kichri is given to all except protovita is given to 6 months to 1 year olds. Lactating mothers are given Kichri/beans out of 7/8 recipies that are locally available-three are must to be chosen. *Births & Deaths 2006-07 :* Live births-62, death-0-1 yr-2 child mortality, 0-5-1. IMR : 32.26 per 1000. CMR : 48.39 per 1000 no MMR : April 06-Jan. 07	Situated opposite the Anganwadi. Pop. of the village as surveyed has *2427* people. Male : 1261—Female : 1166, Children : 0-1 = 61, 1-3 = 110; 3-6 = 185. Dec. 2006, Pregnant mothers—21 to deliver. Generally for vaccination the venue is the Anganwadi centre. Pregnant women 48. They came to sub-centre for weight, Hemoglobin test & blood pressure. High risk mothers-2. Postnatal care women. Visited-7. ANCS—3 examinations refer delivery cases. Like Janani Suraksha yojana, tribal villages have matrutwa anudhan scheme.	They are fisher folk. Two tribals are Hindu Mahadev Koli and Hindu Konkana. They are grape and tomato growers. There is difficulty for drinking water. The whole village was present when we spoke to women. The ex-sarpanch as woman, Nausabai Sukaji Bentkule was articulate and said during three years of her tenure she built a tank for water supply, constructed an auditorium, and homes for the homeless, 2 gram sabha meetings were held in a year but now gram sabha meets 6 times. Drunken men are collectively beaten up by women for becoming a nuisance to the family. **Matrutwa Anudhan** Rs. 800/- as package- of Rs. 400/- in cash is given & for Rs. 400/- protein rich medicines for the pregnant and lactating mother is given.	Some of them were-Vithabai gangurde, Laltha Sanjay Grabhute, Sindhunbai Pawar, Sugandhar M. more Shobov Thete, Pushpa Lahange, Meena Khodade all of them said their mothers had delivery at home and they continue with the practice. She was 28 yrs. Others said had delivery in Mumbai Hospital & had 5 children 3 girls + 2 boys, girls educated upto 8th. After that got operated for family planning. She gets 80 rupees. Sixteen years ago got engaged in agricultural labour. 'Sanji Gobhale 2 : said she has 2 children. Besides 6 yrs. old girl died and four months old boy died of pneumonia. She said she wanted only 2 children. Sugandha married at 15, child at 20 yrs. She treats both equally and educate them. Pushpa married at 16 has 2 girls at home delivery. She is again pregnant. Shobha Thete 32 has 2 children in Nasik civil hospital.

She had *'C'* : section

Women and girls interviewed by me :

51 women, 28 girls, out of them five girls were bold to express what they want in their village. All of them wanted music to be taught in their village.

Rupali wanted a library

Lalita wanted a college

Jyoti wanted 8 posts/for games

Gayatri wanted computer training and

Sujata wanted jim

Bhagyashri a Beauty Parlour.

No food intake is given to lactating mothers

Immediately after delivery, only (tea) chay is given - no milk is given. After 7 days she is given sheera (Rava) Meena Khadade married at 19 yrs. now 22 went for antenatal care to PHC. She also followed what older women practised food intake at home.

Matrutwa Anudhan

This scheme was started to encourage registration of pregnant women, to receive iron and folic acid, vaccination, tonic and four times examination before delivery and will be paid Rs. 100/- for every examination by doctors. (Antenatal care).

High risk cases can be diagnosed, all tests are done, early identification of risk pregnancy and timely referal services provided.

Low weight babies are common- 1 kg to 600 gms

X and breast feeding practices only after a week or 10 days. As in other villages, tribals also believe that by giving milk to the woman after delivery will lead to puss formation which is detrimental to the baby.

Water: Lack of water is a perennial problem in the rocky tribal hills.

Sanitation and hygiene are taken care of by public health that is part and parcel of health system.

Janani Suraksha Yojana

For home delivery, women are given Rs. 500/- for hospital delivery, Rs. 700/- and for *'C'* section, Rs. 1500/- is for non-tribal areas.

Poverty

Another unending misery. But various provisions made by govt. take care of peoples health, education of their children and to some extent provide employment to the youth.

Maharashtra continue

Ambegaon village	*Umroi PHC Sub-Centre in Ambegaon*	*Padas and Padav workers*	*Traditional Birth attendants*	*Weekly list*	*Matrutwa anudhan*
Population : 1545	Shobha V. Thorat ANM : Pathology tests 3rd Monday of every month, Vaccination drive on every Wednesday-Antenatal care clinic is held.	1613 Padav workers are in the district 304 are female workers. There is a proposal to train and turn these padav workers into ASHAs.	Normally called Dais are also encouraged by the Sub-centre to bring pregnant women for institutional delivery. Dais are asked to be with pregnant women at the centre.	Prepared by Padav workers about the name of women, the grade number of issues. Expected date of delivery, name of the village and Pada V (Hamlet).	For BPL this scheme was started for tribal women. Rs. 400/- cash & Rs. 400/- for protein rich medicines for the pregnant women allowed. This is given 4 times at the time of ANC. All pathological tests are made all these efforts and scheme are to encourage institutional deliveries and for mother and child care.
Active Panchayat : **Tara Bai Madhukar Page-Sarpanch of village Panchayat for 2 years now-she got built 2 rooms for the Jilla Parishad Primary school, provided water supply connection and water storage tank for school. Built platform for people to sit in Hanuman Mandir-Assigned cremation ground after consulting the Gramsabha.**	*Meetings of Panchayat* Held Gram Sabha meetings. All people listen to the lady Sarpanch who says she does work sincerely for the good of the community. If I do not work she says, won't people question me as to what I have done? during my tenure. Also she visits sub-centre, school anganwadi and check what quality of nashta is given to children and women.	*Pregnant Women's Mela :* Assistant Child Devept. Project officer has taken the Sarpanch to pregnant women's mela. The lady Sarpanch wanted such a mela for her village and shown this to all villagers. She was interviewed on the AIR—This sarpanch is Hindu Mahadev Koli. Sarpanch acts as counsellor and Advisor to women and her neighbours and women of other villages.	*Sarpanch acquaints women* and people at large about the various schemes and programmes available for the village and its development.	*Birth Register* 39 Births regd. in a year. 25 birth rate per 1000. ANCs regd. are 45. 20 pregnant now & 34 women in labour sent to DT hospital Dindorini. 25 delivered in Community Health Centre, 2 post natal huemmorage treated and Okay.	*Deaths* 9. adults. 0-6. nil. death rate 7.8. no child or infant mortality. No MMR.

Anganwadi Centres

From 300 pop. to 1500, an anganwadi centre is established. ICDS/Tribal development department projects are implemented by the Health department.

Linkage and Convergence

ACDPO when she visits her duty area of ICDS, PHCs and Sub-centres. *Snacks and Mid-day meal.*

Cooked food is served to children and lactating mothers. Shila Ghate is the anganwadi worker.

Family Size & Family Planning

The villagers have got convinced that having small families is good for the health of the family. Hence the women explained that they treat both boys and girls as equal.

Unlike in the urban and non-tribal areas they prefer girls to boys. Since girls do lot of work unlike the men who laze around, drink and play cards.

For undergoing family planning operation women receive Rs. 150/- while men receive Rs. 501.

ANMs-Sub-centres PHCs-CH centres

Women said they lost the knowledge of their parents and ancestors about herbs and medicinal plants. Therefore they have agreed to access medical care for general health and deliveries.

Adoloscent girls receive iron/folic acid tablets once in a week.

Anaemia is the worst malaise amongst women and children.

Kishori Mandals are formed in villages. Lata Jairam Kotwal-12th pass and has done data entry operations. She is awaiting a job.

Education

Educational facilities or vocational training courses are absent in the village.

Facilities for higher education is wanted in the village.

Workload on women

Is high. But they have no empowerment. They suffer the disabilities that women face in other places.

Autonomy

In accessing medi-care in PHCs/Sub-centres or hospitals, group of people of the neighbourhood can take decision about the course of action in labour whether to send the woman to a PHC or sub-centre or a hospital. But the woman has no power to decide about her own delivery.

Maharashtra Continue

Umrale	*Dindori PHC*	*Sub-centres*	*Dr. in charge*	*Anganwadis*
Village population 3400. This village is one kilometer in the interior.	Well equipped with 2 medical officers; both male doctors. 1 male supervisor, 1 lady health worker, ANM-lady pharmacist-1 male lab technician-1 male, driver for jeep. 1 multipurpose worker, 1 sweeper, 4 attendants (1 female + 3 males) for sub-centre 1 ANM-in the Hd. Quarters. Earlier 14 PHCs have been assigned for tribal and 13 for non-tribal areas. Now it has become equal because of the introduction of NRHM.	Seven sub-centres in the PHC area. *Deliveries in PHC* 2006–54 deliveries took place. In the PHC total area has to be perceived as to have had 456 deliveries. *IMR & MMR* 0-1 (13) IMRs in the whole PHC area of 22,463 population 1-5 age group-10 IMR. *ANC* 511 pregnant women have registered & had ante-natal care in the whole area. The register showed 89 women expected to deliver and 50 already delivered.	Dr. P.N. Chavan Medical Officer in charge of PHC. IMR-28.5 for 1000 crude birth rate 20.3 per 1000. Deliveries 40 in the PHC. Referred risk and complicated cases to hospital, 13 out of that 3 cases of C-section. *Family Planning* Regd. cases for sterilisation-tubectomy cases 202. Out of these 190 have been operated upto Jan. 2007. There is a lady health visitor for each PHC area. 6 Bedded PHC with 8 cots were available.	27 anganwadis are there in the PHC area. 27 ANG workers and helpers are appointed. Regularly children and pregnant mothers visit anganwadis where cooked nashta is offered. *Children & Women* lack nutrition. The ANGWs help to arrest this malaise.

Tribal women

Surprisingly tribal women though used to having deliveries at home are queuing up for institutional deliveries in the PHC.

Free medicines and food are given to the women before and after delivery.

Food intake and Breast feeding practises

Suprisingly villages in almost all states follow the practice of not giving milk to the woman who has just delivered. Milk is thought of to produce Puss in the body. The child is not put on breast feeding for 7 to 10 days. Since instl deliveries are taking place, the PHC or sub-centre feed the women with solids and nutritious diet so that the child can gain strength too.

Panchayat

Sarpanch is Krishna Gangorde who is active and Panchas are Bharati Rajendra Bhoye, Pushpa Phagare. At the age of 18 the Sarpanch got married. She has been there for 4 years as sarpanch.

Panchayat meetings are held once in a month.

Leakage in the water supply pipe was repaired. Sarpanch has introduced by her. The adult education. Her husband was farmer Kotwal. After 2 boys and a girl child she got her self operated. Pushpa Phagare herself member who has also 2 girls and a boy got family planning operation done.

Traditional Dais

Four of them are in the village. Happily these dais bring the pregnant women to the centre for delivery and sterilisation. In rare cases where pain starts, Dais themselves attend to the deliveries.

However the concept of milk is not there amongst tribals. They live on roots of plants and on greens grown around.

Training for Anganwadis

Priyanka Pundalik Datrak is an anganwadi worker. Shasikala Rajguru is the supervisor. 60 children visit ANGWs daily without fail. Event 8th pass girls are trained as anganwadis for one full month. Board lodge is provided and group interaction is encouraged. 39–49 ANGWs are there in the more district. 1513 were started this year.

Kishori Shakti Yojana Centers

10% of the girls get counselling are sensitised, on health hygiene, reproductive health, and SHG concept.

This yojana is formed in every Anganwadi Kishori Mandali is for age group from 10th class to 18 years. They are taken as members.

Once they are sensitised, they further are expected to train others.

Kishori

Kishori yojana is to train girls to help anganwadis in distributing iron and folic acid to pregnant women. Young girls are given iron and folic acid too. Once in 2 weeks deworming is done once in 6 months. Their Hemoglobin is also tested.

Andhra Pradesh	Rangareddy dt *All BPL Families*	*Villagers belong to BPL category* *Kesara Mandal* *Kesara I* 890 *M(449) F(441)* *Kesara II* *Pop 607 M 593 F*	*Kesara III* *Pop 965* *484(M) 481(F)*
Education is not a priority though schools upto 10th are there. More infant mortality and less maternal mortality are recorded.	Child labour is rampant, trafficking is a threat mal-nurishment and old archaic ideas that modern medication is poison is still prevalent. Stone crushers are there where women and children work. The superstition is that because their first delivery was normal and at home, they prefer to go to PHCs or hospitals/Pvt. hospitals only for 2nd delivery. Govt./ incentive for girl children if 2nd one is born Rs. 30,000/- is assured for her education and marriage available only at 20 years her age.	Early marriages are common *Errola Sankaramma a young lady got married at 12 and became a mother at 13 years.* When we with a team met her she was working as a voluntary *woman health volunteer* equal to ASHA- who is one per 1000 population, For ANC - Rs. 50/- to be paid to her. Because of ASHA (WHVs) ANMs work load is less here.	Under RCH II WHV are promised more for their services. But no one is paid for BCG—Rs. 25/-, measles—Rs. 50/-, Tubectomy—Rs. 150/-, SC/ST for delivery—Rs. 100/- under Sukhibhava Scheme SCs/STs are promised Rs. 1000 from conception to delivery. Lack of transportation is very much a problem in this area.

Bogaram Village	***Barsaguda Pop. 780 M : F 420-360***	***Vanniguda Pop. 470 M F 247-223***	***Even 0 + 1 infants are taken***
Male domination is there. They drink heavily and beat up women. 20 PHC-8 MTP cases due to WHVs – Women few though come for ANC but no one comes for postnatal check up. Morbidity and lot of problems the women face after delivery. They are afraid to go to PHCs—they never want to visit Sub-centres. For better contractions during delivery they give some *herbal* concentrate. They call it 'Kashayam'. Traditional Dai examines the women in a crude way. Women are kept out in the backyard near cattle shed. Lots of goat rearing is found there. Women and children are anaemic—trends of change is visible. NGOs and SHGs are helping women change their attitudes. Infanticide and foeticide are not uncommon. More abortions are reported.	*Women* tribals drink during pregnancy. They believe that the foetus can move freely in the womb. After delivery also to recoup their strength the women drink. No woman goes to the centre for post-natal checkup. Women face lot of morbidity and lot of problems after delivery. They are afraid to go to PHCs. They never like to go to sub-centres. For better contractions before delivery, women are given 'Kashayam' a herbal concoction. Traditional Dais examine the women in a crude way. Women during and after delivery are kept out in the backyard near cattleshed women and children are anaemic. Infanticide and foeticide are common. NGOs and self help groups are helping woman to change their attitudes. More abortious are reported for girl foetus.	ANMs/WHV are there. They counselled the women - even then for 3 days mothers refuse to feed the babies. Because they believe colostrom is bad and dirty milk not to be fed.	care of by the Anganwadi worker. They believe in Ghosts and at every door-step, chillies are tied to ward off evil spirits.

Renigunta Mandal	*Chittoor district (Royalaseema)*	*Andhra Pradesh*
Chittoor district is one of the backward districts of Andhra Pradesh. Though 100 kms from Chennai, its backwardness is proverbial. Our research team went to Renigunta Mandal PHC and the Villages around : *a BPL area* : 1. Karakambadi 2. Ramakrishnapuram 3. Chaitanya Puram 4. Indira Nagar. We came across low birth weight babies. Discrimination for women labour at work paid Rs. 35/- while men are paid Rs. 60/-, NGO called Rass helps the functioning of the Sub-centres with monetary and physical assistance. Also sponsors education of children and girls.	Social profile poor SCs marriageable age is 12 years to 13 years. Women are sub-servient to men. Drinking by men cause violence on pregnant women and children. Commuting to PHCs to hospitals are difficult for pregnant women.	No easy access to PHC – though PHC is heavily visited by people living around. During pregnancy there are restrictions on food in-take – some fear that children will grow big. 2 cases of maternal mortality is recorded by ANM at PHC. For 3 days the child cannot be breast fed. Honey is given to the baby in drops. Fervent belief in supernatural powers that cause ill health. Women undergo tubectomy, while men refuse family planning devices.

Health Practices of Kumaoni Women Uttarakhand

Modern health care system is concerned with 'medicalisation of life' which according to people of Uttarakhand, takes away the power of the people to heal and take care of themselves. Starting from adoloscence, menstruation to marriage, motherhood, reproductive life, common food eaten by people are avoided. Health according to them is a total way of life integrated to culture and religion, unlike the modern concept of focussing on curing on one to one basis.

Since health, they believe cannot be divorced from their culture and religion, they practise non-medical health measures from menstruation, child birth, rearing of children etc. They do not believe in contraception or vaccination of infants, use of soap or scissors or antibiotics. They have no faith in treatment of water and sewage or insecticide.

Doctors seldom want to work in these rural areas, the hilly regions i.e., : Almorah, Kwedal, Chantala, Kafli.

RCH Survey Report Ramgarh and Dhari Block, Nainital dt.

60 married women, 16/17 age at marriage, 18/19 first pregnancy.

Almorah	*Kwedal*	*Chantala*	*Kafli*
Live births	29— 32	— 10	
Abortions	1 — 2	— 4	IMR is 10 out of 34 births. In Buribaha 6 out of 43 births
Current Pregnant women	3 — 1	— 0	
Infant mortality	0 — 10	— 2	
Born dead	3 — 1	— 2	

Uttaranchal 26/100 (IMR) **(as per charge)**
Garhwal IMR 40/100

After delivery women rest for 11 days. After 22 days women start doing hard work, carry work load – work load is linked to the economic status of the family. Back pain is a common complaint.

Report Sargarhet Clinic

Uttarakhand continued :—

Social and cultural constraints.

Foods avoided by women :

During Menstruation

Milk, curd, mandua Tea with milk, meat, eggs, almonds, garlic. Menstruation is thought as impure. The woman stays in the cattleshed without ventilation. First menstrua-tion after marriage is considered special event for celebration–Pooja performed on the 11th day with 5 elements: dahi, ghee, milk, sesame seeds, and cows urine.

The belif is if any one touches a menstruated woman, will fall sick and develop rashes and can be disastrous to father and brother.

During Pregnancy	Post delivery
Potato,	Corn Chapati
Readish, Rice,	Rice
Lauki ki sabji,	Fried foods
Peanuts	Green vegetables
Walnuts water, Basi	Oily foods
food, Dahi,	Chillies
Onion	

Women are afraid to eat more because they believe the child will grow big and cause difficult delivery.

Both at **Kwedal village** and **Kafli village**, there was no health education and women believed in their superstitious ways.

In **Swukhil village** women after delivery used burnt ash and wrap it up in an old cloth and inserted to soak blood discharge.

Antenatal Practices

Women do not go for antenatal checkup. The family considers as inauspicious.

No check up

Elderly women said pregnancy and delivery are comoon. Why make such fuss of it. We produced seven to eight children; Though 7 died during first two years of birth.

Young mothers cannot over rule mother-in-laws directive and therefore pregnant and lactating mothers avoid pre- and post-natal checkups.

Child birth / delivery		Folk concepts	Child feeding practice
Child birth is ritually polluting while at the same time it is considered auspicious. Purity of the ritual is maintained by the Dai. She does all the rituals only after 22 days women are allowed to cook after purification ceremony of the woman after delivery and havan. Umbilical cord is still to be cut by the mother if not by the mother-in-law who has a right over the health of the child.	Almonds and dates are given to open up the womb Roasted cloves, jaiphal and ghee in milk are given for better contractions during delivery. Methi pani-warm milk are also given for easy contraction. During delivery the Dai presses the vagina of the woman with her foot and heel to stop air going in. The blood that comes out is considered polluting and often hammoerage takes place unttended.	Infant and maternal mortality are punishment by the super-natural for past deeds. If a pregnant woman unduly rests lot, the child in the womb will enlarge leading to difficulty in delivery. After child birth the placenta should be buried under a tree that can bear fruit. This act is considered auspicious.	Traditionally women wait for three to four days to nurse the baby. These women are unaware of the benefits of feeding the baby with cholostram. The woman can rest for 11 days after delivery though she is asked to rest for a month. She has enormous responsibility of maintaining the family. She carries work load and commutes long distances to fetch fuel, fodder and water. The men do not share any household chores to reduce the burden of work on the lactating mother.

Chamoli district

Block Pokhri

Literacy 24 Male/20 Female–

Literacy Male 4 Female 9 –

Villages

Literacy male 45/female 60

Satiana – Population 187 — families — 41 — Male 73 — Female — 114

Hari Shankar — population 225 — families 47, Male 117 — Female —108

Kelab — population — 76 — families 17 — Male 33— Female 43.

Nauta — population — 153 — families 47 — Male 63 — F 90.

Literacy Male 47, female 52

0–6 girl child population is very much less than boys.

HARYANA

Dt. Gurgaon-Block Gurgaon-Village Harsaru

Fact sheet on empirical evidence on socio-eco-determinants behind IMR & MMR.

Population : 2500, Households *450/500,* Male/female *50/50.*

Nearby villages

Gadoli/Sultanpur/Hamirpur/Bamdoli/Dorka/Melka/Dhankot/Bassi/Garhi, Sadrana/Hyatpur etc.

Constraints

For any emergency there is difficulty in finding transport in the nights. Self help group leader volunteers to take women in labour to PHC or civil hospital.

Anganwadis-2

Children from 0-1, 1-3, 3 to 6 are left in the anganwadis though snacks provided to the Anganwadi are for 30/40 children, the swelling numbers to even 80 had to be managed.

Mixed Population

Brahmins, Rajputs and scheduled castes equal numbers. All live in harmony.

Economic Status

Since the area is declared as SEZ, most of the women are landless labourers, construction workers agricultural workers. They are seeking work, they want to earn.

Apprehensive of Doctors

When pregnant women even when they approach private doctors, they are asked to undergo ultra-sound examination, lack of finances prevent the women from above, lack of awareness of civil hospital. Delays in civil hospital-women refuse to go there.

Number of Responsibilities

Anganwadi workers not only attend to children, but also advise mothers on child care, need for vaccination, immunisation, polio drops - about right age of marriage for girls and boys. Keep Birth/death record of pregnant women. Even sometimes record is kept by the chowkidear.

Concerned Departments

Health/family Welfare, Public Health Education, Women and child dept., Rural Development, Panchayat Raj dept. DRDA/Civil Hospital.

Self-help Projects

Women are motivated to form into SH Groups and each contribute Rs. 50/- per month. Once the capital is sizeable. Banks give loans 6 times for women to start productive activity.

Cultural Practices

Older women in the household say they never sought doctors. Delivery is not considered any event special—it is a very ordinary thing to happen—older women help in delivery cases.

Sub-centre—ANM and duties

ANM is expected to be present every day and for the whole day, advise and attend to the needs of pregnant women, ANC and postnatal care-motivate women to seek trained medi-care-keeps Birth/death record.

Concerned Officials and Staff

Deputy Commissioner, Civil Surgeon-Director Health, Director Education Director Women & Child Welfare, Director Public Health/Samiti Council.

Demand by self-help groups

Wants (khaddi) tools for weaving durries - start Dairy farming - buy milking cows/buffaloes and sell milk.

Autonomy-Reproductive Rights of Women

Haryana women are in purdah. Even educated women cannot take decisions about the size of their family/ or for seeking medi-care in PHCs or hospitals. Their mobility is restricted.

Age at time of marriage

Is 18 years for girls and 21 for boys. But most of marriages are for below 16-18 yrs. These are not disclosed—this is the ground truth—the young girls physique does not develop and suit her maternal responsibilities —Result low birth weight babies or death of the infant even maternal mortality is the result also.

Projects

ICDs—Anganwadis PHCs/Sub-centres DRDA/self help groups.

Indira Awas Yojana, Safe motherhood & Child Care Projects, NRH Mission.

Health facilities

Though this is a backward village, may be because it is 10 kms. away from Gurgaon, even sub-centre is not functioning effectively – no PHC, no doctor or nurse. ANM is not there always.

Sex-ratio

Sex-ratio in the state is one of the lowest. Though villagers say boys and girls are equal. Boy preference is evident. In-fanticide in devious ways – practised by older women and Dais.

Age at child birth

Young mothers whose body are mature to deliver babies, she is not aware of child care – she does not attend ante natal care—she does not seek doctors help, may be due to old practices and norms. Maternal mortality cannot be ruled out.

Panchayat

Sarpanch (Lady) Panchas 4 women, Panchas 6 males, Work of Sarpanch handled by male relative. Chandrodevi – Sarpanch.

Traditional Dais

For deliveries they depend on traditional Birth-attendants – since they are not only used to seek her help – but have not much faith in civil hospital.

Birth / Death Registration Compulsory

Anganwadi workers, ANMs, PHCs, Chaukidars, village administrator keep these records. Birth rate/death rates are recorded.

Married/older women workers, AWW/ANM council member – Panchayat President, members, self help groups were interviewed spoken to and observed.

Cultural Practices

Practised even today in the village, food intake for women after delivery – is almost starvation for even 10 to 15 days.

Only tea is given with very little milk because milk is thought of to cause puss formation in the body hence avoided.

No solid food is given only liquids – though after a period of a month or a little earlier she will be fed with ghee (melted butter) and ginger Laddoos etc.

When ajwain is used in any preparation, some one has to guard the woman – same superstition they carry that ajwain (digestive) attracts witches/ bhuths.

Breast feeding practices

Breast feeding of the child is barred for 6 to 10 days or more. People believe that milk will ooze only after the mother takes bath.

The custom that sister-in-law has to arrive at her convenience and then alone the child will be breast fed.

The new born is not allowed to be seen for a few hours even by birth attendants or ANMs/nurses as the case may be.

Child is given ghutti (jaggery water) with a swab, not necessarily sterilised. Child often refuses to suck after getting used to ready made sweet water is given.

Low-birth weight baby

The village women do not believe in keeping the baby in the incubator. They do oil massage to the low birth weight baby also. The rusty blade is used or a kitchen knife is used to cut the umbilical cord.

Patriarchy

Women are totally controlled by men of the family –Even delays take place in risk cases, because-either the husband is not home on time to give permission for taking the women to PHC or civil hospital.

Change

There is a change in outlook towards hospitals and the need to seek medi-care. One has to register for ante-natal care and postnatal care – though the women has no reproductive health rights.She is just a baby delivering machine.

Evidence

Women younger ones spoke of ultrasound machines kept in the mustard fields to avoid penalty/jail term by monitoring civil surgeon and his group of doctors.

Surreptitious behaviour. But ultrasound sex-determination tests are on even today and welcome.

The older women decide the child to be girl if the pregnant women start eating sour things.

They even advise abortion even without undergoing the tests.

Persons/groups of women officials interviewed.

The girls are sent to co-ed primary schools though they do not send them to other villages to pursue higher secondary education for *security reasons they say.*

Infanticide

In confidence one of the doctors revealed that grand mother strangles if the new born is a girl.

MMR

1 lady died immediately 3 hours after delivery in the hospital. Besides medical reasons – there could be socio-economic causes they said.

Remarks

Policies seem remote from ground reality.

The norm used by planners to count only remote villages for grants/funds does not hold good.

It is shocking how such a village almost in the vicinity of the capital is deprived of good health care, half-hearted educational facilities for girls exist.

Nutrition seems no concern for the village women.

Villagers are plying new model cars and motorbikes but their mind-set regarding women, mothers and babies remain unchanged.

BAMDOLI VILLAGE

Population, 2000

Village Bamdoli is 12 kilometers from Gurgaon.

Comparatively urban village lot of construction has been on.

Women appear healthy outwordly—no water problem.

Autonomy

No autonomy is there for women. Even if they are 10th/12th pass, the hold of the mother-in-law/husband is strong.

Their job is to keep the house in order, cook to the orders of the mother-in-law and husband-produce children.

Whether they are older mothers or wives, the men hold the sway, and control women's movement.

Infrastructure

Thee is poor infrastructure.

Households

525 Yadav village 2 Brahmin houses.

Economic Status

Fairly well off families having cattle. Dairies take milk from the village.

Employment

Women do not go out to work. They do not feel the need nor urge to work outside their homes.

Self help groups

No self help group is there. It is thought of as a necessity only for BPL families.

Abortion

Though ANGWs & ANMs are expected to monitor and record - there is only one abortion shown of a woman getting pregnant after 2 months after delivery.

Equal ratio

(First person account) *Age at marriage.*

Sanjokta married at 15 years have three boys-now she is 40.

Suresh 32 years married at 18 yrs, first child at 20. Sona Devi 60-married at 14. 5 children 3 boys and 2 girls.

Birth and death

Sona/girl born at home. died at 1½ months due to phemonia. Boy died on the 5th day.

Murti now 70 + has 4 boys & 1 girl. 3 boys & 3 girls died on 6th day, at 8 months and 6th month. One girl at 15 years died.

Kamla Devi 50 + 6 children-4 girls and 2 boys – one girl died – she was killed.

Krishna Devi 5 deliveries all at home. mother-in-law did not give food after delivery. Sister-in-law steal thing fed me roti/sabji.

Practices

Women were healthy, never went to hospitals nor had abortions nor doctors/nurses visited homes – preferred home deliveries only.

Foods given to women after delivery.

No solid is given, ajwain water, gur given for 10 to 15 days, no milk given fearing it will form into puss and thus harmful to the mother and child—chai is given.

After 15/20 days gradually roti is given not to fill the stomach - only half full is given.

Breast feeding

First infant is given gutti/honey and after 3/4 days allow breast feeding since she will not have milk for 3/4 days to feed.

Never expose the new born even to the nurse/ANM. Only Dai can come and bathe the baby.

Adolescents 115

Yuvashakti programme initiated—ANG worker teaches some crafts to girls and advises on reproductive health. They stop attending school after primary classes.

Fruits banned

Fruits were not given to the lactating mother – now every thing is being given which is not correct say the women of the village.

Method of delivery

Dai alone was the birth attendant. The woman was asked to squat. Deliveries became easier and safer.

No Dais today

After the Dais death no Dai is available in the village. Elderly women now do not want to take any risk.

Seeking medi-care

Not because women have faith in the hospitals but because there are no traditional delivery attendants available. They go to hospitals.

Anganwadi children 53

Visit daily. Poonam-ANG. worker – 10th pass of the same village keeps registers of pregnant women, about birth and deaths.

Nashta

Maize balls are given to children and women – the people desire to receive cooked food that is contemplated and will be furnished soon by the panchayat.

Lack of Knowledge

NRH mission of the Prime Minister is not known to the people in the village. They are unaware of an added functionary called 'ASHA'. Who acts as a bridge between pregnant women and the doctors/PHCs/Sub-centres etc.

Lactating mothers 7 (4+3)

ANM comes once on every 4th week – for attending to vaccination – no one gets checked up by her. Women prefer to go to hospitals in Gurgaon.

Integrated approach

Though the policy is to have a tie up between ANWs and Panchayats, this linkage after gets distorted due to caste differences, ego clashes etc.

Family Planning

Resorted to for women and not men. Women do not want their men to go weak by F.P. operation, older women mother-in-laws do not want their daughter-in-law to go for F.P. She wants more boys in the family.

Pregnant Women 8

If the pregnant women are eating more, older women-decide that the baby will be a girl; they ask women to get the foetus flushed out.

HYATPUR HARIJAN CHAUPAL

Village Sub-centre

Population 1400

Hyatpur is outside Dhani post : Garhi-Harsaru 11 kms from Gurgaon.

Education

Primary school co-education is available. Girls and boys go to school situated in the midst of the village. Older people both male/female are uneducated, without husba-nd's permission we can't send our girls to school they say.

Autonomy

There is no autonomy for women. They are very submissive in this village. They cannot take decision on what to cook, to visit friends or relatives, without permission from in-laws/husband.

Birth/death Registers

Kept by Anganwadis/AWWs/Chowkidars. 6 months ago one case of MMR in the hospital. Her age was 22. She was married at 16 years.

No. of households : 200

Landed and landless labourers. Women do not go out to work. Even if poor, can't go out for work.

Pregnant women

Traditional attendant's services are used. ANM comes to the centre for a short period that too for mere vaccination and distribution of iron and folic acid pills – ANM supposed to keep a register of pregnant women.

Child care

Women marrying at young age are not aware of child care. The women follow their age old practices and beliefs. Anganwadis offer maize balls both to children and lactating mothers.

Self-help group

Hardly any in the village. Even money orders and coming in the name of women can only be received by husbands.

Male/female Ratio : 50 : 50

Though villagers, Sarpanch, ANM and Anganwadis claim of equal sex-ratio, it is far away from the real sex-ratio.

Antenatal and Prenatal care/ Postnatal care

There is no practice of women going for ANC/PN care. Pregnancy is a normal affair and no special event.

Cultural Practices

When a woman whoi's pregnant starts eating sour tamarind/mango, the older women predict that the child to be born will be a girl, quietly abortions are resorted to. Though there is no record kept of abortions by ANMs/ANWs.

Widows : 13-widows

Plight is deplorable. She is thought of as bad omen and not even panchayat comes forward to help them.

PHC 1

9 am-12 noon, one doctor/one nurse/pharmacist (comes 2 days in a week). ANM comes for vaccination.

Ill equipped and villagers and Panchayat seem smug even without having facilities.

Age of marriage

15 to 19 years : *age at child birth* 16 to 18/19 leading to low birth weight babies BPL. Very few BPL no card is issued.

Food habits

Immediately after delivery the mother is almost starved only tea with very little milk is given. Giving milk to drink is believed to cause puss formation, harmful for the woman & child for 10/20 days she is almost starved.

Adult Education

There is no adult education programme in the village nor any other scheme.

	Anganwadis	*Panchayat*	*Environment*	*Public Health*
Traditional Dai-untrained. Attends to 4/5 villages only high risk cases are referred to hospitals mostly private hospitals.	Two in the village. Children 0-1, 1-3 and 3-6 visit and their mothers and pregnant women visit Aganwadis. ANWs have many registers to keep and advise women on vaccination, child care and health.	Sarpanch is a man-Scheduled caste + 3 women of other castes. S.C. people do not co-operate with others in the village. Bharat Singh Sarpanch + 3 women panchas.	Not a clean village drains run through the middle of the galis. Cars/motor cycle run fast in the village.	No contribution of Public Health Department no drainage, no hygiene.

Emergencies

Besides the Dai even ANM/nurse are not available. Risk cases alone are rushed to private hospitals and not to govt. hospital Garhi.

Breast feeding

Child is fed by gutti (sugar/gur in water) with a swab. Mothers milk is not allowed first until sister-in-law comes and washes the breast of the mother and the mother is allowed to breast feed only after she takes bath. Cholestraum is thought of as dirty milk not good for the Baby.

Delays due to

Women in labour and that too in difficult cases hardly reach hospitals on time due to lack of freedom for women to decide and due to lack of available transport specially at night time they are unable to reach Hospitals.

PNDT tests

Available in nearby private clinics are resorted to by well to do mothers - with the permission of in-laws and husband. Haryana has a record low sex-ratio.

Boy Preference

It is common chorus from all women that boys are preferred, but pregnancies continue until boys are born.

Family Planning

No woman is allowed family planning until she delivers boys. Men are not encouraged towards F. Planning. Women feel that their men will go weak after F.P.

Indira Awas Yojana Funds left with DRDA for housing. But conditions stipulated are impractical and thus not implemented.

Why people follow their traditional methods for health care?

1. Women regreted that doctors immediately ask them for ultrasound, check-up-for blood test, we have to go to private doctors. Almost whole day is spent in waiting for prescription and check up in govt. hospitals. Hence we prefer that putting multani mitti (Banni) is good for the health of the child and it is very cooling.
2. For the child we give gutti with honey for a number of days and then alone allow the baby to be breast fed.
3. If there is diarrhoea we give chaval का पानी that stops diarrhoea.
4. We wash our children with atta. This gives them strength and keeps the skin smooth.
5. Medicare is cumbersome for us, it is costly and very time consuming.
6. There is no lady doctor.

There are no self-help groups in the village.

This is a divided village on caste-basis. The scheduled castes wields an upper hand.

No harmony among functionaries

Panchayat is expected to oversee one other *i.e.*, anganwadis, super-anganwadi worker help neither of them meet. ANM is also expected to serve the whole village.

Socially backward

Though economically the villagers appear to be well off, the play of male domination is in full swing. Women are subservient and are totally deprived of decision making.

No Reproductive Child Rights

Women have no right even over the babies in the womb - whether it is abortion, whether to seek medicare, whether to decide the size of her family.

Respondents

Three groups of 20 women each plus Panchayat Sarpanch and members plus ANGs and helpers and Dai plus youth and old.

NRHM

The Panchayat has not heard of the national rural health mission.

ASHA

No one knows who this ASHA is? It is the Panchayat and the ANM in the Panchayat committee appoint/select ASHA a volunteer, who is conceived to act as a bridge between the women and the Hospital/PHC/Sub-centres. If women are in labour, ASHA is expected to take the woman to hospital. Being a volounteer, she is only paid on piece meal work by the beneficiaries and the PHC. There is no ASHA worker.

BPL

There is not even a list of BPL made in the village. 50% of villagers told us that there are people of BPL in the village and others said that there are no BPL.

Security

There is no Police Chowki in the village covering 4/5 villages.

Composition of the Panchayat is multi-caste

While Sarpanch is scheduled caste Shri Bharat Singh. Ayodhya Devi-Panch is of an upper caste, and Rajwati Panch and Savita are other caste members. These women do not happily interact with the sarpanch.

There was no committee meeting held. Now Gram Sabha meetings are held at regular intervals.

Register Keeping

Chowkidar is absent. ANG worker and ANMs register births and deaths. The village administrator issues births and death certificates.

HAMIRPUR VILLAGE

Population 400

Size—Small village populated primarily by Rajputs-Chuhans.

Garhi Village is 5 kms. away but one has to pass through lonely but hescious green fields.

Gurgaon

16 kms. away. This Hamirpur village is a back but not a backward village, though beautifully situated.

Deliveries at Home

Dai lives in Wazirpur attends to deliveries. We have no help in emergencies-no first aid available in the village.

Births/Deaths

Most families have two to 4 children, one of the children 1½ year old reported died of cold.

Male/female : Two : one

Boy Preference

The very ratio reinforces their boy preference to girls.

Much above poverty line

What people need basic infrastructure for providing and supplying water – offering drainage.

Vocational Training

Centre for girls, there is no such centre. Girls educated upto 10th and 12th have no easy access to computer training or colleges.

Distance to hospital

It takes one and half to 2 hours to reach the hospital. Sometimes Gurgaon and at times Garhi.

Households 25

Water

Suffer from lack of water—Personal bore wells only a couple of schedule castes suffer with no water at all.

Panchayat

Wazirpur is the Panchayat that has to look after this village.

Bhupinder Singh Sarpanch +3 women Panchas. Anil is the Panch from Hamirpur.

Primary School Co.-ed.

Education

Only one primary school. Girls want to study further. But parents are insecure to send girls alone to college as the village is reachable after a long tract of aerable fields. One male and one female teacher are appointed.

Most families send their children to Vasant Valley Public School by school bus to Garhi.

Home based provisions

One spoon of honey used to be given to the new born, doctors now don't allow even nipples.

Cholai boiled in salt is given to help child clear bowels.

HAMIRPUR

VILLAGE

Infrastructure

Though affluent a village, it is cut off from the main road. Wazirpur is the nearest village at 2 kms. distance.

No anganwadi is there because of its thin population.

Sub-centre

No sub-centre, no one comes even for administering polio drops.

Wazirpur teacher comes to administer Polio drops.

No rain-water conservation

No governmental infrastructure. Wazirpur Sarpanch does not bother after getting elected.

To the mother

We give gur and ajwain after delivery for 3 days to the mother for 15/20 days, no milk is given to her.

Health Services

No ANM/no one comes for even vaccination of children/pregnant women.

Hygiene and Sanitation

There are no latrines constructed by government. People are not allowed to dig drains.

Road is blocked

Away from the main road the residents owning land do not co-operate to give way for approach road construction.

Indira Awas Yojana

There are 6 BPLs. But only one is allowed a house construction under this yojana.

No facilities for higher education nor for good health/mother and child care.

Girls desirous of pursuing higher studies find it difficult to cross the fields. Panchayat must be able to resolve this mismatch.

Family Planning

Women observed that families have four to five children maximum and there is no need for family planning.

Rich Village

But poor facilities for women and children. No drinking water, no drainage – no latrines – no easy way to cross the village.

SOHNA BLOCK

Bhondse PHC

Population : 7550

Multi Purpose Centre

There is also a oldage home—PHC, anganwadis, play ground.

Panchayat Ghar

PHC, anganwadi, play ground, Vridhashram all situated in the Panchayat Ghar.

Expectant mothers Register is also kept by both Anganwadis and ANHs. They also keeps tab on the condition of pregnant mothers.

April, Dec. 2005 as 139, (no deaths) April-Dec. 2006 as 144-in all.

Register an abortion

Though there is no register kept, their visits to women who are pregnant gives them the feedback.

Households : 983

Building

Huge Building with separate areas for anganwadis and for PHCs.

Emergencies

Women interviewed said they feel safe as pregnant women as delivery hut is started and ANM is always on duty and lives in the village itself.

Women interviewed

About age of marriage Amita, Nirmala, Gita, Rita were vocal and said it varies from 15 to even 19/20 years.

Pregnancies are aborted

Though women openly do not admit abortions sought, they all say it was a miscarriage due to many reasons.

Male/Female Ratio 4/3 : 870 Girls for 1000 Boys

Sohna Block

112 anganwadis, 76 villages and in Bhondse there are 6 anganwadis.

Panchayat's Role

Panchayat's role in safe motherhood and children. Panchayat will now be responsible to arrange cooked food to be distributed to children and women—now increased responsibility.

Age at first Child Birth

Many said 17 years and a few as 20-21 years.

Births/Deaths Jan-Dec. 2005

72 males-8 deaths, 58 females-3 deaths, Jan. to Dec. 2006, 89 males = 151 births 45 deaths in all, 6 boys and 2 girls shown as dead (infants in all).

Concerned Depts.

Health/welfare. Public Health Education, Labour, Rural Development, Panchayat, DRDA, Civil hospital.

Staff in PHC

ANM-Regular, ANM-on contract. Both trained. 1 multipurpose Health worker for immunization, test for malaria, surveys village for population record.

Birth/Death Registers

Records kept both by anganwadi workers and ANMs. The village administrator issues birth certificates of children.

Inference

Male/female sex ratio is questionable since death of males-shown as high and females low, many abortions are not recorded and not reported even.

Projects

ICDS, PHC sub-centres, DRDA/SHGs, Indira Awas Yojana, safe motherhood and child care, NRHM.

Delivery Hut

New experiment started 7 months ago, women use govt./ hospital Sohna or Pvt. doctors—now 10/11 women came to delivery hut every month.

ANM working in close collaboration with anganwadi

Bimla Yadav has to attend to 6 anganwadi area-her salary is 1200/- increment Rs. 100/.

Panchayat

Mahila-Panch never visited anganwadi or PHC.

PHC Bhandse

Well equipped 2 ANMs-one regular Bimla and Sangeeta on contract, she lives in the PHC area attends to women in labour gives medicines.

Autonomy/Reproductive Death

Both newly married/married and older women were interviewed. All agreed that husbands and mothers-in-laws alone have a say even as what to cook, cannot go out even in the village without permission, of course no role for the women to decide the number of children, she would prefer. Until a boy/boys are born, she is expected to go pregnant.

Child Development Programme Officer

Holds 2 meetings in a month with supervisors and anganwadi workers.

Anganwadi

Six in the village atleast more than 60 children come 0-1/1-3 and 3-6.

Traditional Dais

Interviewed two, they said they have no work since women prefer to go to Hospitals/PHCs and dais bring the pregnant women to PHCs.

Anganwadi Supervisor

There are 27 anganwadis in the Sohna Block and supervisor Anupam Hans visits and gives monthly report to CDPO.

PNDT

Tests are on though there is strict monitoring now. Women said compounders keep the ultrasound machines in the fields to avoid detection and punishment.

Anganwadis & women

20/30 women come to anganwadis each day. They are given advice by ANW anganwadi workers. Nashta is given to both children and women dry maize balls. They want cooked food.

Bimla and Meera are Anganwadi workers and Nirmala/Preeti are helpers, Sarla, Premsudha, Shanti all ANW were spoken to in the Bhondse centre.

Family Planning

All women felt men should not go for F. planning, they will became weak.

Alkera

Village

(District Rewari/Block Rewari)

Population : 1650

Economic Status

Many of the households are rich after selling lands and they either remain at home as good housewives.

The landless BPL women have work only for 3 months in a year. Their men work in different vocations throughout the year.

Households : 500

Sex-ratio More Girls than Boys

Sarvasikhsha Abhiyan

Cycles are given to poor Harijan girls to go to school and pursue education upto 11th class.

Village environment

No drainage in the whole village. Comparatively clean village except for the gallis where water stagnates.

Hero Honda helped to get drinking water—sump-pump toilets for girls/boys and teachers are separate in school premises.

Panchayat made one toilet and DRDA model.

Education

Primary school on Roll 174 both boys and girls. 4 male teachers and one lady teacher. Midday meal is provided at 11.30 a.m. Meetha chaval, veg. Pulao, Kichdi, Bakli, Dalia given alternately. The school is upto V class.

Health Check up

Once in 3 months a doctor comes to check up people with difficulties.

ANM visits on every first day of the month. Attends to vaccination, Polio, DPT, etc.

Mahila Mandal

All pregnant and lactating mothers are invited, mostly daughters-in-law are invited. They used to come with their 6 months to 3 year children. Mahila Mandal is discontinued now.

Anganwadi

8.45 a.m. to 12 noon anganwadi functions. Sarla Devi 10th pass is the anganwadi workers. 15 to 20 children at a time are present.

Pre-school education is given to 3 to 4 years olds.

It is situated in the govt. primary school premises. ANG worker. complains that villagers do not co-operate. Shanti Devi is helper.

In all there are 190 anganwadis in Rewari Block.

More than 600 anganwadis in the district.

QUESTIONNAIRE Socio-economic Determinants of IMR (Infant Mortality and Maternal Mortality)

Infant mortality and maternal mortality have not been eliminated in India

Reasons: Can be Medical system, infrastructure, lack of information, awareness, lack of Reproductive rights-no choice, no autonomy for women, poverty, illiteracy, faith in customary practices and beliefs superstition.

Questionnaire:

WHAT ARE THE SOCIO-CULTURAL REASONS FOR INFANT AND CHILD MORTALITY AND MATERNAL MORTALITY.

I. Questionnaires

1. General information of the State/District/Tehsil/ Block/Panchayat/ Village.
2. Geography/Population/Sex-ratio (Male-Female).
3. How many PH centres/CHC (male-female)/Sub-centres are there.
4. How many ANMs are there.
5. Are there doctors posted in the PHC or health centre?
6. Are pregnant women registered by the nurse and Counselled on ante-natal and Post natal Care?

II. Status of the Head of the family/or husband

(a) Name-address etc. Employment.

(b) Is the mother employed?

(c) How many Children born - Survived?

(d) What are the reasons for infant deaths in the family?

(e) How many maternal deaths in the Village?

(f) Are deliveries conducted by untrained/traditional Dais?

(g) Status of hygiene/environment?/delivery place.

III. What are traditional practices

(i) Followed before, during and after delivery?

(ii) In not seeking medical help? What are traditional medicines available?

(iii) In not breast feeding the baby immediately after delivery?

(iv) In not allowing the women to go to health centre or hospital?

(v) Food habits/food intake for the mother and the infant.

(iv) Age at the time of marriage of the Women?

Age at the time of delivery?

How many child births to her and in the family

Any child deaths? at what age?

Are they girls or boys?

What caste/religion of the family?

How do they cause infant deaths and maternal death?

IV. How many Village/block/district level

A. Workers are available? for services and for emergencies?

B. What are your suggestions to improve the situation?

C. Do you suggest change in health policy/Programme/ Scheme?

QUESTIONS-II

To the BDO:	*Revenue Collector*	*Police HD Quarters*	*Health Centres*	*School Teachers*
Composition of your block Bpl families Do they seek Development	Total revenue collected in a year how many land owners?	Are people aware of laws/afraid of Laws/police? How is law and order problem.	Do women seek help from PHCs/ Sub-centres?	how many schools are there? Do girls go to school? Why they drop outs by girls? Do girls marry Young. Do you visit families and advise parents on girls education. Have you stopped child marriages? Do you help panchayats/Anganwadis Do you teach about nutrition.
Occupational Level of people How many Panchayats are there?	How many contractors labourers Are they wage earners?	Clashes between police & people	How many doctors are available? do record of Ancs/ pncs/ deliveries kept/by whom? do pregnant Women get vaccinated? do children get vaccinated? Are medicines given to women Children. Are ANMS available 24 hour	
How many govt. servants? How many Anganwadis Do panchyat members Seek your Advice./	Where do you send the collected revenue?	Do people complain what type? do police stop Caste panchayats. Are cases of kidnapping, human sacrifice, witch hunting, domestic violence, child arriages common?	Who attends in emergencies? Do women prefer DAIs? Do health centres counsel people on health/ hygiene? Are centres well Equipped? Why women are not coming to PHCs/Sub centres?	Are you Secure in the village? As teachers Do you advise People no to believe OJHAs/ Tantrics?
Do people Participate in Activities?	It is spent on health/education. How many govt. schemes are for women?	Do you receive Cases of infanticide, foeticide, PNDT Tests? Dowry demands, Dowry deaths of maternal Mortality?	Is there a change in the mind set of the village.	How do you get water for the
Do people participate in rituals, sacrifices both animal and human. Are children sacrificed to appease the gods and goddesses as advised by tantrics and Ojhas?		Do you allow cultural practices Though Are illegal? Do police also believe in superstition	Are there Records kept of Miscarriages abortions?	In case of rape, Widow remarriage, Inter Caste marriage, does panchyat decide or allow Caste Panchayat to decide? Do panchayat elected members believe in superstition and rituals?

Does Police or Panchayats insist on registration of marriages, infant mortality and maternal mortality?

Why in many villages the chowkidar keeps the register. He is either illiterate or neoliterate.

Does Panchayat chairperson or members interfere in domestic violence, or when a pregnant woman is in need of emergency admission in the hospital or PHCs.

How is it the police does not arrest the older women or the dais who strangle the new born girl child? Is not the police itself is dishonouring the laws?

Since infant mortality and maternal mortality are not merely because of medical or clinical causes, the socio-economic causes and women's lack of empowerment and the hold of the community on the individual life styles are serious determinants.

Are panchayats trained to understand the laws and to honour the laws?

District level household facility and survey on reproductive and child health (Rd 2, 2002-4) Sponsored by: (Ministry of Health & Family Welfare) Govt. of India, New Delhi

Haryana	*Tamil Nadu*	*Andhra Pradesh*	*Rajasthan*	*Maharashtra*	*Uttarakhand*
Antenatal checkup	ANC	ANC	ANC	ANC	ANC
87.6	99.4	94.5	68.1	92.9	62.6
Delivery by Skilled Persons					
43.2	89.2	69.0	44.4	62.6	32.5
Full immunization					
62.9	92.1	62.9	25.4	74.3	47.2
Current use of any family planning methods					
60.3	57.7	62.8	46.9	63.3	48.7
Unmet needs					
14.7	18.1	11.7	21.8	12.6	26.9
Adequately staffed PHCs					
59.3	72.9	64.8	28.00	78.4	40.5

Percentage of PHCs adequately equipped in

States *Care Kit*	*Birth order*	*Ranking*	*Infra-structure*	*Staff*	*Supply*	*Equipment*	*Training*	*E.D.*
Haryana	38.4	21	54.6	59.3	46.2	41.2	50.4	28.2
Rajasthan	47.4	31	33.2	28.0	69.2	53.9	14.8	36.1
Uttaranchal	45.9	24	27.8	40.5	23.6	27.1	7.6	13.2
Maharashtra	32.4	12	76.5	78.4	67.4	91.4	31.9	48.7
Tamil Nadu	21.6	4	64.7	72.9	77.8	92.2	27.7	14.4
Andhra Pradesh	22.5	13	59.2	64.8	40.3	84.5	34.5	34.5

District level household facility and survey on reproductive and child health (Rd 2, 2002-4)

Girls Marriage below age	*Haryana*	*Mean age at Boys*	*Marriage Girls*	*Current Use of Contraception*	*Modern method*	*Condom*	*(Unmet need) Limiting*	*Spacing*
18	27.8%	22.7	19.0	60.3%	54.4%	10%	9.2%	5.5%
18	Rajasthan							
	49.4%	20.6	17.3	46.9%	42.3%	6.2%	13.7%	8.1%
18	Uttaranchal							
	9.8%	24.6	20.5	48.7%	44.2%	11.1%	17.1%	9.8%
18	Maharashtra							
	21.1%	24.6	19.1	63.3%	60.8%	4.9%	7.1%	5.5%
18	Tamil Nadu							
	15.5%	26.4	20.7	57.7%	55.0	2.1%	12.7%	5.4%
18	Andhra Pradesh							
	38.6	23.2	18.4	62.8	62.4	0.4	6.1	5.6

States	*ANC (Percent)*			*Delivery Percent)*			*Immunization (Percent)*		*Percent Received ORS*	
	Atleast 1 TT injection	*Recd. IFA tablets*	*Full ANC*	*Govt. Insti-tution*	*Home*	*Attended by skilled person*	*Injections of DPT*	*Measles*	*Full*	*ORS%*
Haryana	85.8%	17.1%	11.8	10.6	64.8	43.2	75.7	69.2	62.9	32.1
Rajasthan	69.0%	8.0	5.0	19.4	68.0	44.4	36.4	36.8	25.4	29.4
Uttaranchal	71.2%	20.0	10.5	10.7	76.2	32.5	57.7	56.9	47.2	21.4
Maharashtra	90.9%	28.1	23.0	24.1	41.7	62.6	88.5	88.0	74.3	42.0
Tamil Nadu	97.4	24.7	23.5	44.5	13.4	89.2	96.8	95.7	92.1	35.8
Andhra Pradesh	87.9	48.3	43.9	22.1	38.6	69.0	78.7	74.4	62.9	58.6

MONITORABLE TARGETS FOR THE TENTH PLAN AND BEYOND

- Reduction of poverty ratio by 5 percentage points by 2007 and by 15 percentage points by 2012;
- Providing gainful and high-quality employment at least to addition to the labour force over the Tenth Plan period;
- All children in school by 2003; all children to complete 5 years of schooling by 2007;
- Reduction in gender gaps in literacy and wage rates by at least 50 per cent by 2007;
- Reduction in the decadal rate of population growth between 2001 and 2011 to 16.2 per cent;
- Increase in Literacy rates to 75 per cent within the Plan period;
- Reduction of Infant mortality rate (IMR) to 45 per 1000 live births by 2007 and to 28 by 2012;
- Reduction of Maternal mortality ratio (MMR) to 2 per 1000 live births by 2007 and to 1 by 2012;
- Increase in forest and tree cover to 25 per cent by 2007 and 33 per cent by 2012;
- All villages to have sustained access to potable drinking water within the Plan period;
- Cleaning of all major polluted rivers by 2007 and other notified stretches by 2012.

Midterm Review/Planning Commission

Discussions in Parliament

[Shri R. Ramakrishnan] Aircraft [RAJYA SABHA]

7. Shri Hukmdeo Narayan Yadav
8. Shri Rameshwar Singh
9. Shri Dipen Ghosh
10. Shri Nepaldev Bhattacharya
11. Shri Hari Shankar Bhabhra
12. Shrimati Mohinder Kaur
13. Shri Kalraj Mishra
14. Prof. Sourendra Bhattacharjee
15. Shri Shiva Chandra Jha

with instructions to report by the first week of the next session."

The motion was negatived.

THE VICE-CHAIRMAN (SHRI R. RAMAKRISHNAN): I shall now put the motion of Shri Khurshed Alam Khan to vote. The question is;

"That the Bill further to amend the Aircraft Act, 1934, be taken into consideration."

The motion was adopted.

THE VICE-CHAIRMAN (SHRI R. RAMAKRISHNAN): We shall now take up clause by clause consideration of the Bill.

Clauses 2 and 3 were added to the Bill Clause 1.
Short Title

SHRI KHURSHED ALAM KHAN: Sir, I beg to move:

"That at page 1, line 3, *for* the figure "1982" the figure "1983" be *substituted.*"

The question was put and the motion adopted.

THE VICE-CHAIRMAN (SHRI R. RAMAKRISHNAN): The question is:

"That Clause 1, as amended, stand part of the Bill."

The motion was adopted.

"Clause I as amended, was added to the Bill."

Enacting formula (Amdt.) Bill, 1982

SHRI KHURSHED ALAM KHAN: Sir, I beg to move:

"That at page 1, line 1, *for* the word "Thirty-third" the word "Thirty-fourth" be *"substituted."*

The question was put and the motion was adopted.

THE VICE-CHAIRMAN (SHRI R. RAMAKRISHNAN): The question is:

"That the Enacting Formula, as amended, stand part of the Bill."

The motion was adopted.

"The Enacting Formula as amended, was added to the Bill."

The Title was added to the Bill.

SHRI KHURSHED ALAM KHAN: Sir, I move:

"That the Bill, as amended, be passed."

The question was put and the motion was adopted.

HALF-AN-HOUR DISCUSSION ON POINTS ARISING OUT OF THE ANSWER GIVEN IN THE RAJYA SABHA ON THE 23RD FEBRUARY, 1983, TO STARRED QUESTION 43, REGARDING INFANT MORTALITY RATE IN THE COUNTRY.

THE VICE-CHAIRMAN (SHRI R. RAMAKRISHNAN): Now, we shall take up half-an-hour discussion.

DR. M.M.S. SIDDHU (Uttar Pradesh): No statistics express better the difference between a society of sufficiency and a society of deprivation than the infant mortality rate. It is particularly sensitive to the distribution of resources. It reflects not only the per capita stock of food, clean water, medical care, etc. but the actual availability to all segments of the population. Deprivation of the people in a particular region, class or group is likely to show up in the infant mortality rate.

Sir, as the figures given out in the Health Statistics of India, 1981, show the picture of the infant mortality rate from the years 1970 to 1978 is not very encouraging. Rather, I will say, it is depressing. In 1970, the combined infant mortality rate was 129 and in the year 1978 it is 125. In other words, we have been able to save 4 lives per thousand. But if we were to analyse the rural and the urban, in the rural one, 136 is the rate in 1970 but in 1978 it is 136. In other words, there has been no improvement in reducing the infant mortality rate in the rural areas. And you will find a greater disparity between the rural and urban. In rural sector it is 136 and in the urban sector it is 90, nearly 80 per cent of what it was in 1970. And there has been a good fall in the year 1978. It has been reduced to 70. From 90 to 70 has been the reduction in the infant mortality rate in urban areas. But in the rural areas, we have not been able to reach the expectant mother.

Sir, when we come to male and female ratio, again we will find that males die less as compared to females. When we come to another age Group, we find again, as far as rural areas are concerned, it is left untouched in the age group of '0 to 4'. In 1970, it was 55.5; in 1971, it was 55.3; and in 1976, it was 54.2. But the female rate as compared to the male is higher—55.5 to 61.0. And the same is the case in the urban areas. In that age group of 0 to 4, for male, it was 32.3 in 1970 and 29.0 in 1976. Sir, these statistics only reveal that female children die more as compared to the male children. And secondly the disparity between the rural and urban areas, the gap between the two is much more and is increasing.

Sir, the reasons which were given by the hon. Minister were: first; the prematurity. As far as prematurity is concerned, it is a well-known fact that prematurity is caused by early birth and low birth weight. The factors which affect adversely the survival rate of the new born are : naternal age place of delivery low socio-economic status, inadequate pre-natal nutrition, heavy physical work during pregnancy, inter-uterine infection alcoholic consumption and smoking. Most of them are such which are preventive.

The other reasons which have been stated are birth injury and intrauterine asphyxia. They are mostly related to accoucheuse or the working of the birth attendant. I will come to this point later on whether the dais who are being trained are sufficient in number. The other reason which has been stated is tetanus. Well, Sir, when we think of immunisation programme as a preventive inoculation of the mother which protects as well the newborn, according to the Report of Ministry of Health for 1981-82, about 7.9 million expectant mothers were to be inoculated or prevented by tetanus oxide, and the achievement was expected to be 70 per cent. The total births in a year are about 21 million. The actual persons immunized is 5-3 million. It works out to 25 per cent of the total figure or one-fourth of the mothers are protected and three fourths are left outside the immunisation programme. How to reach them is the main question? And again if you were to break it in terms of rural and urban, this immunisation programme is mostly urban rather than rural. Sir, it has also been said that diarrhoeal diseases, infection and malnutrition were the main causes of the rise in infant mortality. The two major factors which contribute to the present state of health of children are under-nutrition resulting from inadequate diet, infection and insanitary involvement. Well, Sir, as far as malnutrition is concerned, it is effected in two ways. Every child in a poor family suffers from repeated bouts of diarrhoea and in the course of years the child undergoes a decline in health and the nutritional status falls. *(Time Bell rings)*. Sir, I will take, a couple of minutes more I will take' two or three minutes. I won't make more time. When the nutritional status falls, the oral dehydration therezy help in acute stage. But in the case of chronic diarrhoea, it does not help but the education of the mother and secondly, the potable water supply. These two factors not being there, the education being faulty and the chronic infection along with it leads to low protein diet and malnutrition. Then, again, Sir, as far as the child's diet is concerned, it has to be improved. We have the integrated programme of nutrition. But according to Dr. Gopalan, former Director of the ICMR "The latest data show that from the child surveyed only in 40 per cent of cases diets had been considered adequate. The situation is similar to what has been reported nearly 20 years ago." It is estimated, according to him, that 45 million children of the pre-school age in our country subsist on inadequate diet. The answer is not only to give them 300 calories that they get from the integrated pre-school programme, which is not even half the diet that they required, that is about 1200 calories. So, the daily intake of these children is low.

Sir, as far as the infrastructure is concerned, all that I can say is that I will 'only read what has been publish-ed in the official journal "Swastha" In March-April 1981 issue, where a survey has been made in Rajasthan and the conclusion is that the service rendered by the primary health centres and sub-centres failed to meet the expectation of the people. It goes on to say, Sir, that where the sub-centres are concerned which have been recommended as one of the major breakthrough by which infant mortality will be reduced, this is what the author has to say "All the sub-centres reminded eligible couples to maintain registers but no sub-centre had an uptodate register. The number of deliveries conducted by the sub-centre staff varied from one to two in a month. But in quite a few centres no delivery was conducted by the sub-centre staff during the last five years." This being the state of affairs all the infrastructure of the sub-centres which we are building, I have nothing more to say except that the monitoring and implementation is bad and an evaluation should be lone. (*Time Bell rings*).

Sir, I am coming to the last point. Sir, the Nutrition Institute of Hyderabad had conducted some of the studies in urban households as to how our education programme of health goes on and it was revealed that among the low income groups the percentage of listeners to the radio instructional broadcast was very poor; unattractive bland representation was one of the important reasons." Sir, now we come to the question how we can reduce infant mortality in our country. I would like to give the example of Kerala.

The Vice-Chairman (Shri R. Ramakrishnan)

Please conclude; because time is short three more speakers are there and we have to adjourn at 6.

DR. M. M. S. SIDDHU

I will take one or two minutes. Sir, in Kerala the *per capita* income at the time of the study in 1980 was low as compared to Punjab. The expenditure on primary health care was more and nutrition supply from the fair-price shops was better than in Punjab. And thus they reduced the infant mortality rate to 50 per cent. That is how priorities have to be given.

Therefore, the programme that has been enunciated in the reply will not meet the requirement of reducing infant mortality even to the level of Sri Lanka which is 50 per thousand births, what to talk of developed countries where it is 8 to 10 per thousand births.

The Minister of Health and Family Welfare (Shri B. Shankaranand)

Mr. Vice-Chairman, the hon. Member, who himself is a doctor and a very knowledgeable person in field of health and other matters relating to this country, has given all facts and figures. I need not go into all these; I have got with me facts, figures and the data but since you have said that you are going to adjourn at 6 and there are three more speakers, I would be brief.

I do say that the Government is very seriously concerned with this problem of infant mortality. We have not been able to make much progress in cutting down this death rate which grapples the infant either at the pre-natal stage or the pari-natal stage.

The hon. Member referred to the question of health of the school-going children. Of course, it would take some time to explain about the school-going children, because we have taken school health programme and other matters, as the hon. Members are aware of it. So, instead of going into the details, I do agree that as per the data that is available, infant mortality in rural areas, amongst illiterate masses and poor families is more. We have not been able to do much to cover the rural population As can be seen from the activities I have enunciated more often than once in this House and in the other House, the health infrastructure that has been built up in these years, especially in the Sixth Five Year Plan has been so large that we have been trying to cover as large a population as possible, and this can be seen from the measures that we have taken that an elaborate infrastructure has been built in this country consisting of 6042 primary health centres, 65,000 sub-centres, 2500 urban family welfare centres, 550 post-partum entres, 341 paediatric. Units, especially in the district hospitals, and 24 sick new-born units have been started. These are receiving the support of our 4 lakh trained dais, 23 lakh village health guides, 66,700 trainers and 13,800 LHVs. Besides these, more than 450 primary health centre doctors have been given special training in MCH and 29 professors of paediatrics from medical colleges have been attending besides demonstration of paediatrics curriculum and 32 professors have been integrated with the MCH family planning programme. I am quoting it because these are the things that we have taken up. You know, to achieve results, it takes time. It is not the case that today we have got this infrastructure and results should come tomorrow. The results of this will be seen over a couple of years. The hon. Member has mentioned about the immunisation programme. We have increased the coverage of the programme and this immunisation programme is against DPT, TT, Diarr hoea and other things. I can give the figures for the last three years, from 1979-80 to 1981-82. This is the number of beneficiaries we have been able to cover. I am quoting the number. DPT—22.38 million, Polio—4.16 million, TT for pregnant mothers—16.37 million and nutritional anaemia cases—13 million. This has been the coverage during the last three years from 1979-80 to 1981-82.

I do agree with the hon. Member that it is not only medical intervention or providing health infrastructure to the people which can cut down the infant mortality rate. It has to be coupled with health education. We have enough, health education material for the health educators at the level of village health guides, *dais,* ANMs, LHB and primary health centres and sub-centres. This is basically to educate the expectant mothers and others in the society. It is this sort of education which will prevent and cut down the infant mortality rate in the rural areas.

This is a phenomenon which cannot be tickled by mere medical intervention, by merely providing the services and supplies. This has to be dealt with in relation to the overall eeconomic development of the people as a whole. This is a socio-economic phenomenon. People should be made aware of environmental sanitation, personal hygiene and so on. The economic standards, the living standards, education, literacy, all these things go a long way in solving the problem. It is not the task of the Health Ministry alone. We have an inter-sectoral approach in this regard. The minimum needs programme which has been taken to the rural areas is going to help us in a long way in giving the people proper nutrition, proper purchasing power, in raising the living standards of the people and in giving them a sense of well-being. This is going to help us in reducing the infant mortality rate. We have been trying our best. I have given the figures. We will be able to produce the expected results in a couple of years.

श्री शिव चन्द्र झा (बिहार) : उप-सभाध्यक्ष महोदय, इनफेंट मार्टेलिटी रोकने में जो कदम हों उनमें एक जरूरी कदम मैं समझता हूं कि खासकर रूरल एरियाज में देहाती इलाकों में जहां कि 75-80 प्रतिशत लोग रहते हैं, गांव की बनावट आइडियल हो। सरकार के सामने आइडियल, विलेज की योजना हो जिसमें कि पीने का पानी सफाई और साथ ही साथ गड्ढे रहते हैं उनको ठीक करें आइडियल विलेज बनाना शुरू हो देहात में तो मैं समझता हूं कि इनफेंट मार्टेलिटी का रेट कम होगा और बच्चे जो मर जाते हैं खराब पानी की वजह से वह रूक जाएगा। तो मैं सरकार से जानना चाहता हूं कि इसके लिए आइडियल विलेज बनाने की योजना अपकी है या नहीं?

दूसरा, न्यूर्टिशस फूड देने के लिए क्या योजना है। कहीं-कहीं तो शायद आज दिया भी जाता है, लेकिन जिनको मिलना चाहिए उनको न मिल कर जिनको नहीं मिलना चाहिए उनको मिलता है या जो इंचार्ज है वही हड़प जाते हैं। क्या आपको इसका कुछ पता है और इसमें सुधार करेंगे? तीसरा और आखिरी सवाल मेरा यह है कि अब तक इनफेंट मार्टेलिटी को रोकने के लिए आपने कितना पैसा खर्च किया? पहली योजना से लेकर पांचवी योजना तक कितना पैसा खर्च किया और 6ठीं योजना में कितना पैसा अलाट किया गया है? यह मेरे सवाल है जिनका जवाब मैं चाहता हूं।

SHRI SHRIDHAR WASUDEO DHABE (Maharashtra): Sir, the Minister in his statement has said that the majority of these deaths are not due to malnutrition. About 69 per cent are due to other reasons. That means at least 31 per cent deaths are due to malnutrition. May I know from the hon. Minister whether there is any programme of midday meals for the school-going children In the Centrally-administered areas? It is the direct responsibility of the Central Government. In some States this midday meals programme is being executed, but I would like to know if it is going to be there in the schools of the Centrally-administered areas.

Secondly, one of the reasons for these deaths is that there are untrained birth attendants (dais) in rural areas. Is there, any programme for, training these birth attendants, parit-i cularly in the rural areas or in the slum ! areas? These dais are paid very nominally these days a'hd that is one of the reasons which goes to increase the mortality rate. These are" my two questions.

SHRI B. SHANKARANAND: Sir hon. Shiva Chandra Jha has asked about the provisions in the Fifth Plan and other Plans. I have got a long list of these things and I can lay it on the Table of the House for the information of the hon. Members. *(Interruptions)*. As I have said earlier, It is not only the provision for immunisation and some such other things, but it is the expenditure which is spread to various branches for raising the living standards and which ultimately goes to raising the status of the people which will ultimately help in cutting down the infant mortality. So to give a total figure of expenditure is very difficult.

Regarding the question of Shri Dhabe about the mid-day meals programme, it is not the concern of the Health

Ministry, but I should say that the Social Welfare Ministry is having some programme for the benefit of the nursing mothers and children. This is the programme being monitored by the Social Welfare Ministry and the mid-day meal programme is not the concern of the Health Ministry, we do' not come into the picture there.

श्री शिव चन्द्र झा: आइडियल विलिज की कोई योजना है या नहीं? इसमें माइंड की बात नहीं है। नक्शा भी है। एक्सपेरीमेंट भी हो रहा है।

उप-सभाध्यक्ष (श्री आर. रामकृष्णन) जवाब दे दिया है।

SHRI B. SHANKARANAND: Ideal village is in everybody's mind.

SHRI SHRIDHAR WASUDEO DHÀBE: Any programme for training of *dais*?

SHRI B. SHANKARANAND: The hon. Member should know that there is a programme for elementary education, adult education, rural health, water supply, rural roads, rural electrification, house sites, houses for rural landless labourers, environmental improvement of slums and nutrition. If this programme is properly implemented it will go a long way in establishing the rural life and an ideal life. Regarding registration of *dais,* there is nothing like registration of *dais.* We have trained *dais* and the target is that we will train one dai for every one thousand population and we hope to cover the entire population by the end of 1984.

THE VICE-CHAIRMAN (SHRI R. RAMAKRISHNAN): The Half-an-Hour Discussion is concluded and the House stands adjourned till 11.00 am tomorrow.

The House adjourned at fifty-nine minutes past five of the clock till eleven of the clock on Wednesday, the 16th March, 1983.

MATERNAL MORTALITY RATIO
(per 1,00,000 live births)

	1997-98	*1999-01*	*2001-03*
India	**398**	**327**	**301**
Andhra Pradesh	197	220	195
Assam	568	398	490
Bihar	531	400	371
Gujarat	46	202	172
Haryana	136	176	162
Karnataka	245	266	228
Kerala	150	149	110
Madhya Pradesh	441	407	379
Maharashtra	166	169	149
Orissa	346	424	358
Punjab	280	177	178
Rajasthan	508	501	445
Tamil Nadu	131	167	134
Uttar Pradesh	606	539	517
West Bengal	303	218	194

INFANT MORTALITY RATE (IMR)

Sl. No.	*States*	*2000*	*2001*	*2002*	*2003*	*2004*	*2005*
	ALL INDIA	**68**	**66**	**63**	**60**	**58**	**58**
1.	Andhra Pradesh	65	66	62	59	59	57
2.	Assam	75	74	70	67	66	68
3.	Bihar	62	62	61	60	61	61
4.	Chhattisgarh	79	77	73	70	60	63
5.	Gujarat	62	60	60	57	53	54
6.	Haryana	67	66	62	59	61	60
7.	Jharkhand	70	62	51	51	49	50
8.	Karnataka	57	58	55	52	49	50
9.	Kerala	14	11	10	11	12	14
10.	Madhya Pradesh	87	86	85	82	79	76
11.	Maharashtra	48	45	45	42	36	36
12.	Orissa	95	91	87	83	77	75
13.	Punjab	52	52	51	49	45	44
14.	Rajasthan	79	80	78	75	67	68
15.	Tamil Nadu	51	49	44	43	41	37
16.	Uttar Pradesh	83	83	80	76	72	73
17.	West Bengal	51	51	49	46	40	38
18.	Himachal Pradesh	60	54	52	49	51	49
19.	J&K	50	48	45	44	49	50
20.	Arunachal Pradesh	44	39	37	34	38	37
21.	Delhi	32	29	30	28	32	35
22.	Goa	23	19	17	16	17	16
23.	Manipur	23	20	14	16	14	13
24.	Meghalaya	58	56	61	57	54	49
25.	Mizoram	21	19	14	16	19	20
26.	Nagaland	NA	NA	NA	NA	17	18

27.	Sikkim	49	42	34	33	32	30
28.	Tripura	41	39	34	32	32	31
29.	Uttaranchal	50	48	41	41	42	42
30.	A&N Islands	23	18	15	18	19	27
31.	Chandigarh	28	24	21	19	21	19
32.	D&N Haveli	58	58	56	54	48	42
33.	Daman & Diu	48	40	42	39	37	28
34.	Lakshadweep	27	33	25	26	30	22
35.	Pondicherry	23	22	22	24	24	28

Source: Sample Registration System, Registrar General, India.

Women's health and development, related indicators India

Indicator		*Latest available data*	*Year*	*Source*	*Remarks*
1. COUNTRY SITUATION					
Population and vital statistics					
Total population (in millions)		846.3[a]	1991	1	
Population growth rate (%)		1.6	1995-2000	2	Projection
Urban population (%)		25.7[a]	1991	1	
Population density (per sq km)		291	1997	3	
Average household size	Urban	4.7	1987-88	4	
	Rural	5.1	1987-88	4	
Crude birth rate (per 1000 population)		28.3	1995	5	
Crude death rate (per 1000 population)		9.0	1995	5	
Under-five mortality rate (per 1000 live births)		90	1997	6	
Singulate mean age at first marriage (years)					
	Female	20.0	1992-93	7	
	Male	25.0	1992-93	7	
Marriage rate (per 1000 population)					
	Total	496	1994	8	
	Female	544	1994	8	
	Male	451	1994	8	

Indicator		*Latest available Data*	*Year*	*Source*	*Remarks*
Urban	Female[c]	464	1991	1	
Rural	Female[c]	482	1991	1	
Divorce rate (per 1000 population)		7.41	1991	1	
Socio-economic situation					
GNP per capita (US $)		370	1997	9	
Per cent of GDP from agriculture (at 1980-81 prices)		27.91	1995	10	
Per cent of population below poverty line[e]					
	Total	36.0	1993-94	10	
	Urban	32.4	1993-94	10	
	Rural	37.3	1993-94	10	
Per cent of GDP spent on					
Health and family welfare (at current prices)		2.5	1995-96	10	
Education, art, culture and youth affairs (at current prices)		3.93	1995-96	10	
Defence[f]		2.57	1996-97	10	

Sources

1. Ministry of Public Health. *DPR Korea country report on the second evaluation of the implementation of the health for all strategy.* Pyongyang; 1990.
2. Ministry of Public Health. *DPR Korea country report on the third evaluation of the implementation of the health for all strategy.* Pyongyang; 1997.
3. United Nations. *World population prospects: the 1996 revision.* New York: Oxford University Press; 1996.
4. United Nations Development Programme. *Human development report 1997.* New York: Oxford University Press; 1997.
5. United Nations. *The world's women 1995: trends and statistics.* New York: United Nations; 1995.
6. Inter-Parliamentary Union. *Men and women in politics: democracy in the making.* Geneva: Inter-Parliamentary Union; 1997.
7. Data reported to World Health Organization on maternal mortality estimates, World Health Organization, Regional Office for South-East Asia, New Delhi, India; 1998.
8. United Nations Development Programme. *Human development report 1996.* New York: Oxford University Press; 1996.
9. Women of south-east Asia (A Health Profile) (WHO).
10. Regional Publications SEARO, No. 34, New Delhi, 2000.

Chart No. 5

INFANT MORTALITY RATE IN INDIA

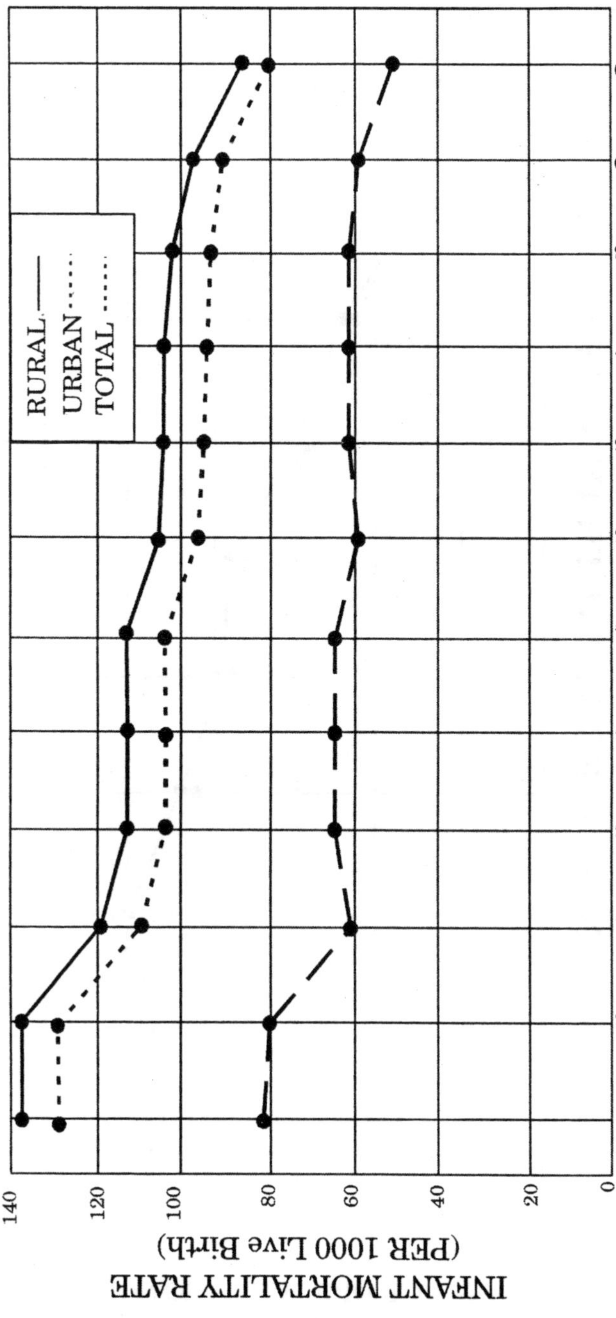

Chart No. 7
EXPECTATION OF LIFE AT BIRTH IN YEARS 1901-1990

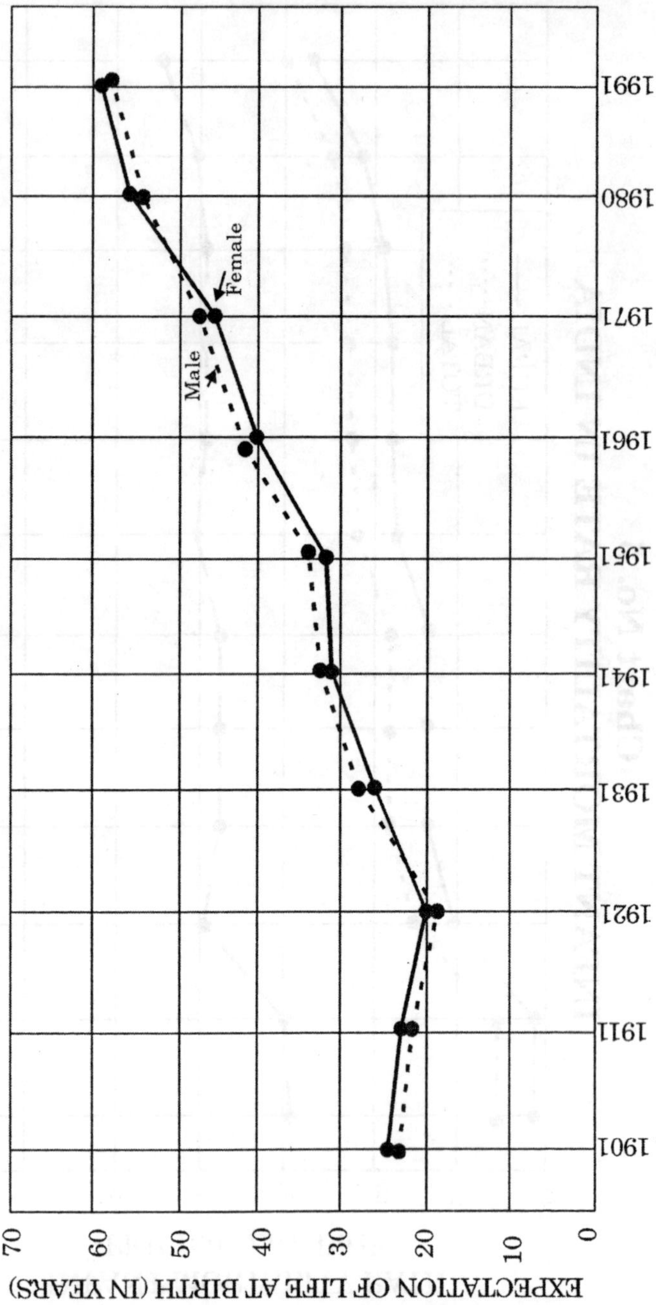

VOLUME 34 NO. 2 OCTOBER 2000

SAMPLE REGISTRATION SYSTEM BULLETIN

Published Bi-Annually in April and October Each Year—ISSN 0971-3549

REGISTRAR GENERAL, INDIA

Vital Statistics Division, West Block 1, Wing 1, 2nd Floor, R.K. Puram, New Delhi-110 066

Sample Registration Bulletin which used to be published in July and January is now being published three months earlier in April and October respectively in a new concise format. This effort will facilitate faster dissemination of the SRS results to all the data users. The October issue presents the provisional figures for 1999.

Table 1 gives the provisional estimates of birth rate, death rate and infant mortality rate for India, States and Union territories for the year 1999. Table 2 gives the estimates of birth rate, death rate and infant mortality rate for India. States and Union territories for the latest three years 1996-1998 for comparative reference.

Table 1. Provisional estimates of Birth rate, Death rate, Natural growth rate and Infant mortality rate, 1999

India / States / Union Territories	*Birth rate*			*Death rate*			*Natural growth rate*			*Infant mortality rate*		
	Total	*Rural*	*Urban*	*Total*	*Rural*	*Urban*	*Total*	*Rural*	*Urban*	*Total*	*Rural*	*Urban*
1	*2*	*3*	*4*	*5*	*6*	*7*	*8*	*9*	*10*	*11*	*12*	*13"*
India*	**26.1**	**27.6**	**/20.8**	**8.7**	**9-4**	**6.3**	**17.3**	**18.2**	**14.5**	**70**	**75**	**44**
Bigger States												
1. Andhra Pradcsh	21.7	22.0	20.6	8.2	9.0	5.7	13.5	13.1	15.0	66	75	37

	1	*2*	*3*	*4*	*5*	*6*	*7*	*8*	*9*	*10*	*11*	*12*	*13"*
2.	Assam	27.0	28.0	18.9	9.7	10.1	6.2	17.3	17.9	12.7	76	79	36
3.	Bihar	30.4	31.3	22.6	9.1	9.3	6.6	21.4	22.0	16.0	66	67	51
4.	Gujarat	25.4	27.0	22.0	7.9	8.8	5.9	17.6	18.2	16.1	63	70	45
5.	Haryana	26.8	27.7	23.3	7.7	8.0	6.4	19.1	19.7	16.9	68	70	58
7.	Karnataka	22.3	23.7	19.2	7.7	8.7	5.5	14.6	15.0	13.6	58	69	24
8.	Kerala	18.0	18.1	17.7	6.4	6.5	6.3	11.5	11.6	11.4	14	14	16
9.	Madhya Pradesh	30.7	32.1	23.4	10.6	11.2	7.4	20.1	20.9	15.9	91	96	55
10.	Maharashtra	21.1	21.6	20.3	7.5	8.7	5.6	13.6	12.9	14.7	48	58	31
11.	Orissa	24.1	24.6	20.3	10.6	11.1	7.1	13.4	13.5	13.3	97	100	65
12.	Punjab	21.5	22.5	18.6	7.4	7.9	6.1	14.1	14.6	12.5	53	57	39
13.	Rajasthan	31.1	32.5	24.9	8.4	8.9	6.4	22.7	23.6	18.5	81	85	59
14.	Tamil Nadu	19.3	19.8	18.2	8.0	8.7	6.6	11.3	11.1	11.6	52	58	39
15.	Uttar Pradesh	32.1	33.1	26.7	10.5	11.0	7.7	21.6	22.1	19.0	84	87	64
16.	West Bengal	20.7	22.9	14.3	7.1	7.2	6.8	13.6	15.7	7.5	52	55	40
Smaller States													
1.	Arunachal Pradesh	22.3	23.2	13.5	6,0	6.4	1.9	16.3	16.7	11.6	43	45	10
2.	Goa	14.3	14.4	14.1	7.2	7.6	6.6	7.1	6.8	7.5	21	23	17
3.	Himachal Pradesh	23.8	24.3	16.8	7.3	7.5	5.2	16.4	16.8	11.6	62	63	38

1	2	3	4	5	6	7	8	9	10	11	12	13"
4. Manipur	18.6	19.4	16.4	5.4	5.0	6.6	13.1	14.3	9.8	25	22	24
5. Meghalaya	28.7	31.1	15.7	9.1	10.2	3.3	19.5	20.9	12.4	56	59	33
6. Mizoram	17.0	18.7	14.8	5.5	6.9	3.7	11.5	11.8	11.1.	19	22	14
7. Nagaland	N.A.	N.A.	11.8	N.A.	N.A.	2.3	N.A.	N.A.	9.5	N.A.	N.A.	16
8. Sikkim	21.6	21.9	14.7	5.8	5.9	3.4	15.8	16.0	11.3	49	50	33
9. Tripura	17.0	17.5	14.4	5.7	5.7	5.7	11.3	11.8	8.7	42	43	33
Union Territories												
1. Andaman & Nicobar Islands	18.1	17.8	19.2	5.5	6.2	3.5	12.6	11.5	15.7	25	30	9
2. Chandigarh	17.9	24.5	17.1	3.9	2.6	4.1	14.0	21.9	13.0	28	36	27
3. Dadra & Nagar Haveli	32.4	35.2	23.5	5.9	7.0	2.3	26.5	28.1	21.2	56	61	7
4. Daman & Diu	26.9	24.9	28.8	7.1	8.9	5.4	19.9	16.1	23.3	35	34	36
5. Delhi	19.4	20.7	19.3	4.8	4.5	4.9	14.6	16.2	14.4	31	33	31
6. Lakshadweep	25.1	25.1	25.0	4.7	4.3	5.0	20.4	20.8	20.0	32	26	37
7. Pondicherry	17.7	18.0	17.5	6.9	7.9	6.1	10.8	10.1	11.4	22	32	15

* : Excludes Nagaland (Rural) & Jammu & Kashmir due to part-receipt of returns.
N. A.: Not available due to part-receipt of returns.
Note : Infant mortality rates for Smaller States and Union Territories are for the period 1997-99.

With compliments from Jayant Kumar Banthia, Registrar General, India, 2-A Mansingh Road, New Delhi-110 011, India.
Phones : E-mail : rgindia @ hub.nic.in ((91) (11) 338 3761 Fax : (91) (11) 338 3145
Census and Vital Statistics Website on the Internet : http://www.censusindia.net

VOLUME 35 NO. 2 OCTOBER 2001

SAMPLE REGISTRATION SYSTEM BULLETIN

Published Bi-Annually in April and October Each Year—ISSN 0971-3549

REGISTRAR GENERAL, INDIA

Vital Statistics Division, West Block 1, Wing 1, 2nd Floor, R.K. Puram, New Delhi-110 066

Table 1. Provisional estimates of Birth rate, Death rate, Natural growth rate and Infant mortality rate, 2000

India / States / Union Territories	*Birth rate*			*Death rate*			*Natural growth rate*			*Infant mortality rate*		
	Total	*Rural*	*Urban*	*Total*	*Rural*	*Urban*	*Total*	*Rural*	*Urban*	*Total*	*Rural*	*Urban*
1	*2*	*3*	*4*	*5*	*6*	*7*	*8*	*9*	*10*	*11*	*12*	*13*
India*	**25.8**	**27.5**	**20.7**	**8.5**	**9.3**	**6.3**	**17.3**	**18.3**	**14.4**	**68**	**74**	**43**
Bigger States												
1. Andhra Pradesh	21.3	21.7	20.1	8.2	9.0	5.8	13.1	12.7	14.3	65	74	36
2. Assam	26.9	27.9	18.6	9.6	10.0	6.1	17.4	17.9	12.6	75	78	35
3. Bihar	31.9	32.8	25.6	8.8	9.1	7.1	23.1	23.7	18.5	62	63	53
4. Gujarat	25.2	26.8	21.9	7.5	8.3	5.8	17.7	18.4	16.1	62	69	45
5. Haryana	26.9	27.9	23.0	7.5	7.9	6.2	19.4	20.1	16.7	67	69	57
7. Karnataka	22.0	23.3	19.1	7.8	8.6	5.7	14.2	14.6	13.3	57	68	24

	1	*2*	*3*	*4*	*5*	*6*	*7*	*8*	*9*	*10*	*11*	*12*	*13"*
8.	Kerala	17.9	18.0	17.5	6.4	6.5	6.2	11.5	11.6	11.4	14	14	14
9.	Madhya Pradesh	31.2	33.2	23.5	10.2	11.0	7.5	21.0	22.2	16.1	88	94	54
10.	Maharashtra	20.9	21.2	20.3	7.5	8.6	5.7	13,4	12.7	14.6	48	57	33
11.	Orissa	24.3	24.8	20.1	10.5	11.0	7.0	13.7	13.8	13.1	96	99	66
12.	Punjab	21.5	22.6	18.5	7.3	7.8	5.8	14.2	14.8	12.6	52	56	38
13.	Rajasthan	31.2	32.6	25.0	8.4	8.8	6.5	22.8	23.7	18.5	79	83	58
14.	Tamil Nadu	19.2	19.9	18.0	7.9	8.6	6.4	11.3	11.2	11.5	51	57	38
15.	Uttar Pradesh	32.8	34.0	27.2	10.3	10.8	8.0	22.5	23.2	19.1	83	87	65
16.	West Bengal	20.6	23.0	14.0	7.0	7.1	6.7	13.6	15.8	7.3	51	54	37
Smaller States													
1.	Arunachal Pradesh	22.3	23.1	13.9	6.0	6.3	2.5	16.3	16.8	11.4	44	45	11
2.	Chhatisgarh	26.7	29.2	22.8	9.6	11.2	7.1	17.1	18.0	15.7	79	95	49
3.	Goa	14.3	14.3	14.2	7.4	7.9	6.7	6.8	6.4	7.5	23	24	21
4.	Jharkhand	26.5	28.8	19.4	9.0	9.8	6.5	17.6	19.0	13.0	70	74	48
5.	Himachal Pradesh	22.1	22.5	16.9	7.2	7.3	5.5	14.9	15.2	11.4	60	62	37
6.	Jammu & Kashmir	19.6	20.3	16.5	6.2	6.3	5.9	13.4	14.1	10.6	50	51	45
7.	Manipur	18.3	19.1	16.2	5.6	5.4	6.0	12.7	13.6	10.2	23	23	25
8.	Meghalaya	28.5	31.0	15.3	9.2	10.1	4.6	19.3	20.9	10.7	58	61	32

1		2	3	4	5	6	7	8	9	10	11	12	13"
9.	Mizoram	16.9	18.8	14.5	5.2	6.3	3.7	11.7	12.6	10.7	21	24	15
10.	Nagaland	N.A.	N.A.	12.2	N.A.	N.A.	3.0	N.A.	N.A.	9.2	N.A.	N.A.	23
11.	Sikkim	21.8	22.1	14.8	5.7	5.7	4.0	16.2	16.4	10.7	49	49	36
12.	Tripura	16.5	17.0	14.0	5.4	5.3	5.6	11.1	11.6	8.4	41	42	32
13.	Uttaranchal	20.2	24.6	17.1	6.9	10.3	4.5	13.3	14.3	12.6	50	73	26
Union territories													
1.	Andaman & Nicobar Islands	19.1	19.0	19.3	5.1	5.7	3.4	14.0	13.3	15.9	23	27	10
2.	Chandigarh	17.5	18.9	17.3	3.9	3.8	3.9	13.6	15.1	13.4	28	38	26
3.	Dadra & Nagar Haveli	34.9	35.9	24.0	7.8	8.2	3.5	27.0	27.7	20.4	58	62	14
4.	Daman & Diu	23.7	21.8	25.4	6.6	7.1	6.2	17.1	14.7	19.2	48	38	57
5.	Delhi	20.3	21.4	20.1	5.1	5.0	5.1	15.1	16.4	15.0	32	32	32
6.	Lakshadweep	26.1	27.6	24.6	6.0	7.1	4.9	20.1	20.5	19.7	27	25	29
7.	Pondicherry	17.8	18.4	17.4	6.5	7.2	6.0	11.3	11.2	11.3	23	33	15

* : Excludes Nagaland (Rural) due to part-receipt of returns.

N. A.: Not available due to part-receipt of returns.

Note : Infant mortality rates for Smaller States and Union Territories are for the period 1998-2000.

With compliemnts from Jayant Kumar Banthia, Registrar General, India, 2-A Mansingh Road, New Delhi-110 011, India.
E-mail : orgindia @vsnlnet Phone : ((91) (11) 338 3761 Fax : (91) (11) 338 3145
Census and Vital Statistics Website on the Internet : http://www.censusindia.net

Table 2. Estimates of birth rate, death rate and infant mortality rate for the latest three years, 1997-1999

India / States / Union Territories	*Year*	*Birth rate*			*Death rate*			*Infant mortality rate*		
		Total	*Rural*	*Urban*	*Total*	*Rural*	*Urban*	*Total*	*Rural*	*Urban*
1	*2*	*3*	*4*	*5*	*6*	*7*	*8*	*9*	*10*	*11*
India *1997	**27.2**	**28.9**	**21.5**	**8.9**	**9.6**	**6.5**	**71**	**77**	**45**	
	1998	**26.5**	**28.0**	**21.0**	**9.0**	**9.7**	**6.6**	**72**	**77**	**45**
	1999	**26.0**	**27.6**	**20.8**	**8.6**	**9.4**	**6.3**	**70**	**75**	**44**
Bigger States										
1. Andhra Pradesh	1997	22.5	23.1	20.5	8.3	9.1	5.9	63	70	37
	1998	22.4	22.8	20.9	8.8	9.7	6.0	66	75	38
	1999	21.7	22.0	20.6	8.2	9.0	5.7	66	75	37
2. Assam	1997	28.2	29.0	20.7	9.9	10.3	5.9	76	79	37
	1998	27.9	28.7	20.2	10.0	10.5	6.0	76	80	36
	1999	27.0	28.0	18.9	9.7	10.1	6.2	76	79	36
3. Bihar	1997	31.7	32.7	23.6	10.0	10.4	6.8	71	73	53
	1998	31.1	32.1	23.1	9.4	9.7	6.5	67	68	51
	1999	31.5	32.4	25.2	8.9	9.2	7.1	63	64	55

1	2	3	4	5	6	7	8	9	10	11
4. Gujarat	1997	25.6	27.0	22.6	7.6	8.3	6.2	62	69	46
	1998	25.5	27.0	21.9	7.9	8.6	6.3	64	71	46
	1999	25.4	27.0	22.0	7.9	8.8	5.9	63	70	45
5. Haryana	1997	28.3	29.6	23.8	8.0	8.3	6.9	68	70	59
	1998	27.6	28.8	23.2	8.2	8.6	6.8	70	72	59
	1999	26.8	27.7	23.3	7.7	8.0	6.4	68	70	58
6. Karnataka	1997	22.7	23.9	20.1	7.6	8.5	5.4	53	63	24
	1998	22.0	23.1	19.4	7.9	8.9	5.6	58	70	25
	1999	22.3	23.7	19.2	7.7	8.7	5.5	58	69	24
7. Kerala	1997	17.9	17.9	17.9	6.2	6.3	6.1	12	11	15
	1998	18.3	18.3	18.0	6.4	6.5	6.2	16	15	17
	1999	18.0	18.1	17.7	6.4	6.5	6.3	14	14	16
8. Madhya Pradesh	1997	31.9	33.6	23.1	11.0	11.7	7.7	94	99	57
	1998	30.7	32.1	23.0	11.2	11.9	7.8	98	104	56
	1999	31.1	33.1	23.6	10.4	11.1	7.6	90	96	55
9. Maharashtra	1997	23.1	24.4	21.0	7.3	8.6	5.4	47	56	31
	.1998	22.5	23.6	20.4	7.7	8.9	5.6	49	58	32
	1999	21.1	21.6	20.3	7.5	8.7	5.6	48	58	31

1		2	3	4	5	6	7	8	9	10	11
10.	Orissa	1997	26.5	27.2	21.3	10.9	11.3	7.5	96	100	65
		1998	25.7	26.4	20.9	11.1	11.6	7.6	98	101	66
		1999	24.1	24.6	20.3	10.7	11.1	7.1	97	100	65
11.	Punjab	1997	23.4	24.9	19.0	7.4	7.8	6.1	51	54	38
		1998	22.4	23.7	18.5	7.7	8.2	6.3	54	58	40
		1999	21.5	22.5	18.6	7.4	7.9	6.1	53	57	39
12.	Rajasthan	1997	32.1	33.7	25.1	8.9	9.3	7.0	85	89	61
		1998	31.6	33.1	24.6	8.8	9.3	6.9	83	87	60
		1999	31.1	32.5	24.9	8.4	8.9	6.4	81	85	59
13.	Tamil Nadu	1997	19.0	19:3	18.3	8.0	8.7	6.7	53	58	40
		1998	19.2	19.7	18.1	8.5	9.3	6.8	53	59	40
		1999	19.3	19.8	18.2	8.0	8.7	6.6	52	58	39
14.	Uttar Pradesh	1997	33.5	34.6	27.9	10.3	10.7	8.2	85	89	66
		1998	32.4	33.4	27.2	10.5	10.9	8.1	85	89	65
		1999	32.8	33.9	27.5	10.5	11.1	8.1	84	88	66
15.	West Bengal	1997	22.4	24.8	15.9	7.7	7.9	7.2	55	58	43
		1998	21.3	23.4	15.2	7.5	7.7	7.1	53	56	41
		1999	20.7	22.9	14.3	7.1	7.2	6.8	52	55	40

1	2	3	4	5	6	7	8	9	10	11
Smaller States										
1. Arunachal Pradesh	1997	21.4	22.3	12.2	5.8	6.1	2.0	47	49	17
	1998	22.5	23.3	13.6	6.1	6.5	1.8	44	46	10
	1999	22.3	23.2	13.5	6.0	6.4	1.9	43	45	10
2. Chhatisgarh	1997	Included in Madhya Pradesh								
	1998	Included in Madhya Pradesh								
	1999	26.9	29.3	23.6	9.6	11.3	7.0	78	95	47
3. Goa	1997	14.2	14.4	13.8	7.7	8.0	7.2	19	23	14
	1998	14.3	14.6	13.8	8.2	8.5	7.7	23	25	22
	1999	14.3	14.4	14.1	7.2	7.6	6.6	21	23	17
4. Jharkhand	1997	Included in Bihar								
	1998	Included in Bihar								
	1999	26.3	28.5	19.0	8.9	9.7	6.4	71	76	48
5. Himachal Pradesh	1997	22.6	23.1	16.8	8.1	8.3	5.9	63	64	38
	1998	22.6	23.0	16.9	7.7	7.9	5.4	64	66	38
	1999	23.8	24.3	16.8	7.3	7.5	5.2	62	63	38
6. Jammu & Kashmir	1997	Not available due to part-receipt of returns								
	1998	19.8	20.8	15.8	5.4	5.6	4.4	45	46	44
	1999	20.9	22.0	16.5	6.3	6.2	6.3	52	53	44

1		*2*	*3*	*4*	*5*	*6*	*7*	*8*	*9*	*10*	*11*
7.	Manipur	1997	19.7	20.5	17.6	5.9	5.8	6.2	30	31	28
		1998	19.0	19.9	16.7	5.3	5.1	6.1	25	22	26
		1999	18.6	19.4	16.4	5.4	5.0	6.6	25	27	24
8.	Meghalaya	1997	30.2	32.9	16.6	8.8	9.7	4.4	54	56	52
		1998	29.2	31.8	15.6	9.0	9.9	4.2	52	54	36
		1999	28.7	31.1	15.7	9.1	10.2	3.3	56	59	33
9.	Mizoram	1997	15.0	16.4	13.3	4.8	5.7	3.7	19	22	15
		1998	15.8	18.1	13.1	5.6	6.7	4.3	23	26	18
		1999	17.0	18.7	14.8	5.5	6.9	3.7	19	22	14
10.	Nagaland	1997	N.A	N.A	7.9	N.A	N.A	2.7	N.A.	N.A	16
		1998	N.A	N.A	11.9	N.A	N.A	1.7	N.A	N.A	16
		1999	N.A	N.A	11.8	N.A	N.A	2.3	N.A	N.A	16
11.	Sikkim	1997	19.8	20.0	12.8	6.5	6.6	3.5	51	51	41
		1998	20.9	21.2	13.5	6.1	6.2	3.9	52	52	44
		1999	21.6	21.9	14.7	5.8	5.9	3.4	49	50	33
12.	Tripura	1997	18.3	18.9	15.5	6.8	6.9	5.8	51	53	39
		1998	17.6	18.2	14.8	6.1	6.2	5.4	49	50	39
		1999	17.0	17.5	14.4	5.7	5.7	5.7	42	43	33

1	2	3	4	5	6	7	8	9	10	11
13. Uttaranchal	1997	Includedin UttarPradesh								
	1998	Included in Uttar Pradesh								
	1999	19.6	24.5	16.1	6.5	10.5	3.5	52	75	27
Union Territories										
1. Andaman & Nicobar Islands	1997	18.6	18.8	17.8	5.1	5.6	3.6	33	39	16
	1998	17.7	18.0	16.8	4.6	5.1	3.0	30	37	9
	1999	18.1	17.8	19.2	5.5	6.2	3.5	25	30	9
2. Chandigarh	1997	18.8	20.9	18.5	4.2	3.7	4.3	40	46	40
	1998	17.9	21.3	17.5	4.1	3.5	4.2	32	44	30
	1999	17.9	24.5	17.1	3.9	2.6	4.1	28	36	27
3. Dadra & Nagar Haveli	1997	28.2	28.7	22.8	8.2	8.6	3.6	63	67	7
	1998	34.1	35.1	23.4	7.9	8.4	3.0	61	65	7
	1999	34.2	35.2	23.6	6.6	7.0	2.5	56	61	7
4. Daman & Diu	1997	24.9	25.5	24.4	5.9	7.7	4.4	38	41	35
	1998	21.7	23.0	20.5	7.0	8.1	6.1	51	42	59
	1999	26.9	24.9	28.8	7.1	8.9	5.4	35	34	36
5. Delhi	1997	21.1	22.7	20.9	5.4	5.4	5.4	35	34	35
	1998	19.4	20.9	19.3	5.3	5.3	5.3	36	36	36
	1999	20.3	20.7	20.3	4.8	4.5	4.9	31	33	31

1		2	3	4	5	6	7	8	9	10	11
6.	Lakshadweep	1997	22.9	23.5	22,3	6.2	6.1	6.3	36	22	49
		1998	23.0	23.5	22.3	6.2	6.1	6.3	26	22	30
		1999	25.1	25.1	25.0	4.7	4.3	5.0	32	26	37
7.	Pondicherry	1997	18.4	20.1	17.1	8.0	9.1	7.2	22	30	16
		1998	18.2	18.3	17.9	7.8	8.7	7.2	21	31	14
		1999	17.7	18.0	17.5	6.9	7.9	6.1	22	32	15

* Excludes Jammu & Kashmir for the year 1997 due to part-receipt of returns.

N.A. Not available due to non-receipt of returns.

Note: Infant mortality rate for smaller states/UT's shown against 1997, 1998 and 1999 are for the periods 1995-97. 1996-98 and 1997-99 respectively.

About the Sample Registration System (SRS)

The Sample Registration System (SRS) is a large scale demographic survey for providing reliable annual estimates of birth rate, death rate and other fertility and mortality indicators at the national and sub-national levels. The vital rates for 1999 in respect of the three newly created states of Chhatisgarh, Jharkhand and Uttaranchal were presented in the April, 2001 issue of SRS bulletin. The present issue also contains the vital rates for 2000 for these states. The field investigation consists of continuous enumeration of births and deaths by a resident part time enumerator, generally a teacher and an independent survey every six months by a computer supervisor. The data obtained through these operations are matched. The unmatched and partially matched events are re-verified in the field and thereafter an unduplicated count of births and deaths is obtained. The SRS was initiated by the OFFICE OF THE REGISTRAR GENERAL, INDIA on a pilot basis in a few selected states in 1964-65 and it became fully operational during 1969-70 with about 3700 sample units. Thereafter the number of sample units was periodically increased. The sample unit in rural areas is a village or a segment of it if the village had a population of 1500 or more. In urban areas the sampling unit is a census enumeration block with a population ranging from 750 to 1000. At present SRS has 6671 sample units (4436 rural and 2235 urban) in all States and Union territories covering about 1.1 million households and 6.28 million population.

SRS BULLETIN
SAMPLE REGISTRATION SYSTEM
REGISTRAR GENERAL, INDIA
Vital Statistics Division, West Block 1, Wing 1, 2nd Floor, R.K. Puram, New Delhi-110 066

Table 1. Estimated Birth rate, Death rate, Natural growth rate and Infant mortality rate, 1999

India / States / Union Territories	*Birth rate*			*Death rate*			*Natural growth rate*			*Infant mortality rate*		
	Total	*Rural*	*Urban*	*Total*	*Rural*	*Urban*	*Total*	*Rural*	*Urban*	*Total*	*Rural*	*Urban*
1	*2*	*3*	*4*	*5*	*6*	*7*	*8*	*9*	*10*	*11*	*12*	*13*
India	**26.1**	**27.6**	**20.8**	**8.7**	**9.4**	**6.3**	**17.4**	**18.2**	**14.5**	**70**	**75**	**44**
Bigger States												
1. Andhra Pradesh	21.7	22.0	20.6	8.2	9.0	5.7	13.5	13.1	15.0	66	75	37
2. Assam	27.0	28.0	18.9	9.7	10.1	6.2	17.3	17.9	12.8	76	79	36
3. Bihar	31.5	32.4	25.2	8.9	9.2	7.1	22.6	23.2	18.	63	64	55
4. Gujarat	25.4	27.0	22.0	7.9	8.8	5.9	17.6	18.2	16.	63	70	45
5. Haryana	26.8	27.7	23.3	7.7	8.0	6.4	19.1	19.7	16.9	68	70	58
6. Karnataka	22.3	23.7	19.2	7.7	8.7	5.5	14.6	15.0	13.6	58	69	24
7. Kerala	18.0	18.1	17.7	6.4	6.5	6.3	11.5	11.6	11.4	14	14	16

1		2	3	4	5	6	7	8	9	10	11	12	13
8.	Madhya Pradesh	31.1	33.1	23.6	10.4	11.1	7.6	20.7	21.9	15.9	90	96	55
9.	Maharashtra	21.1	21.6	20.3	7.5	8.7	5.6	13.6	12.9	14.7	48	58	31
10.	Orissa	24.1	24.6	20.3	10.7	11.1	7.1	13.4	13.5	13.2	97	100	65
11.	Punjab	21.5	22.5	18.6	7.4	7.9	6.1	14.1	14.6	12.5	53	57	39
12.	Rajasthan	31.1	32.5	24.9	8.4	8.9	6.4	22.7	23.6	18.5	81	85	59
13.	Tamil Nadu	19.3	19.8	18.2	8.0	8.7	6.6	11.3	11.1	11.6	52	58	39
14.	Uttar Pradesh	32.8	33.9	27.5	10.5	11.1	8.1	22.2	22.9	19.4	84	88	66
15.	West Bengal	20.7	22.9	14.3	7.1	7.2	6.8	13.6	15.7	7.5	52	55	40
Smaller States													
1.	Arunachal Pradesh	22.3	23.2	13.5	6.0	6.4	1.9	16.3	16.7	11.6	43	45	10
2.	Chhatisgarh	26.9	29.3	23.6	9.6	11.3	7.0	17.4	18.0	16.5	78	95	47
3.	Goa	14.3	14.4	14.1	7 2	7.6	6.6	7.1	6.8	7.5	21	23	17
4.	Jharkhand	26.3	28.5	19.0	8.9	9.7	6.4	17.4	18.9	12.6	71	76	48
5.	Himachal Pradesh	23.8	24.3	16.8	7.3	7.5	5.2	16.4	16.8	11.6	62	63	3S
6.	Jammu & Kashmir	Data not complied due to part-receipt of return											
7.	Manipur	18.6	19.4	16.4	5.4	5.0	6.6	13.2	14.3	9.8	25	22	24
8.	Meghalaya	28.7	31.1	15.7	9.1	10.2	3.3	19.5	20.9	12.4	56	59	33
9.	Mizoram	17.0	18.7	14.8	5.5	6.9	3.7	11.5	11.8	11.1	19	22	14

	1	*2*	*3*	*4*	*5*	*6*	*7*	*8*	*9*	*10*	*11*	*12*	*13*
10.	Nagaland	11.8	N.A.	11.8	2.3	N.A.	2.3	9.5	N.A.	9.5	N.A	N.A	16
11.	Sikkim	21.6	21.9	14.7	5.8	5.9	3.4	15.8	16.0	11.3	49	50	33
12.	Tripura	17.0	17.5	14.4	5.7	5.7	5.7	11.3	11.8	8.7	42	43	33
13.	Uttaranchal	19.6	24.5	16.1	6.5	10.5	3.5	13.2	14.0	12.5	52	75	27
Union Territories													
1.	Andaman & Nicobar Islands	18.1	17.8	19.2	5.5	6.2	3.5	12.6	11.5	15.7	25	30	9
2.	Chandigarh	17.9	24.5	17.1	3.9	2.6	4.1	14.0	21.9	13.0	28	36	26
3.	Dadra & Nagar Haveli	34.2	35.2	23.6	6.6	7.0	2.5	27.5	28.1	21.0	56	61	7
4.	Daman & Diu	26.9	24.9	28.8	7.1	8.9	5.4	19.9	16.0	23.3	35	34	36
5.	Delhi	20.3	20.7	20.3	4.8	4.5	4.9	15.5	16.2	15.4	31	33	31
6.	Lakshadweep	25.1	25.1	25.0	4.7	4.3	5.0	20.4	20.8	20.0	32	26	37
7.	Pondicherry	17.7	18.0	17.5	6.9	7.9	6.1	10.8	10.1	11.4	12	32	15

N. A.: Not available due to part-receipt of returns.

Note : Infant mortality rates for Smaller States and Union Territories are for the three-year period 1997-99 for Mizoram it is for 1997-99.

With compliments from Jayant Kumar Banthia, Registrar General, India, 2-A Mansingh Road, New Delhi-110 011, India.
E-mail : rgindia and hub.nic.in @ ((91) (11) 338 3761 Fax : (91) (11) 338 3145
Census and Vital Statistics Website on the Internet : http://www.censusindia.net.

India/States/ Union Territories	Birth Rate						Death	
	Total		Rural		Urban		Total	
	Lower Limit	Upper Limit	Lower Limit	Upper limit	Lower limit	Upper Limit	Lower limit	Upper limit
1	2	3	4	5	6	7	8	9
India	**25.9**	**26.3**	**27.3**	**27.8**	**20.4**	**21.3**	**8.6**	**8.8**
Bigger States								
1. Andhra Pradesh	21.1	22.3	21.4	22.7	19.3	21.9	7.8	8.6
2. Assam	25.8	28.3	26.6	29.3	17.1	20.8	8.7	10.7
3. Bihar	30.8	32.3	31.6	33.2	23.1	27.3	8.6	9.3
4. Gujarat	24.5	26.3	25.9	28.1	20.4	23.7	7.5	8.3
5. Haryana	25.7	27.9	29.8	32.5	21.1	25.5	7.1	8.2
6. Karnataka	21.5	23.3	22.7	24.7	17.5	20.9	7.4	8.1
7. Kerala	17.4	18.5	17.5	18.6	16.3	19.1	6.1	6.7
8. Madhya Pradesh	30.2	32.1	31.9	34.2	21.9	25.3	10.6	11.7
9. Maharashtra	20.3	21.9	20.8	22.4	18.8	21.8	7.1	7.8
10. Orissa	23.3	24.9	23.7	25.5	18.8	21.9	10.1	11.2
11. Punjab	20.7	22.3	21.5	23.4	17.1	20.1	7.0	7.8
12. Rajasthan	30.2	32.1	31.4	33.5	23.3	26.6	8.0	8.9

1	2	3	4	5	6	7	8	9
13. Tamil Nadu	18.7	19.9	19.1	20.5	17.1	19.3	7.7	83.4
14. Uttar Pradesh	32.2	33.4	32.2	34.7	26.1	28.8	10.2	10.8
15. West Bengal	20.0	21.3	22.2	23.6	13.2	15.4	6.8	7.3
Smaller States								
1. Arunachal Pradesh	17.7	26.9	18.0	28.3	9.9	17.2		
2. Chhatisgarh	25.3	28.5	27.8	30.7	20.0	27.2		
3. Goa	13.2	15.4	13.1	15.8	12.2	15.9		
4. Jharkhand	25.0	27.5	27.1	30.0	16.4	21.6		
5. Himachal Pradesh	22.3	25.2	22.8	25.9	14.8	18.7		
6. Jammu & Kashmir			Not available					
7. Manipur	14.6	18.2	0.0	0.0	14.6	18.2		
8. Meghalaya	24.8	32.6	26.4	35.8	11.5	19.9		
9. Mizoram	14.7	19.2	16.1	21.4	10.9	18.6		
10. Nagaland	N.A.	N.A.	N.A.	N.A.	7.4	16.2		
11. Sikkim	10.5	19.0	0.0	0.0	10.5	19.0		
12. Tripura	16.0	17.9	16.7	18.3	10.2	18.6		
13. Uttaranchal	18.3	20.9	22.0	27.0	14.4	17.8		

Union Territories							
1.	Andaman & Nicobar Islands	16.3	19.9	16.1	19.4	14.2	24.1
2.	Chandigarh	15.1	20.7	15.7	33.4	14.1	20.1
3.	Dadra & Nagar Haveli	29.5	35.3	32.1	38.3	19.3	27.7
4.	Daman & Diu	22.5	31.3	22.9	26.9	21.9	35.6
5.	Delhi	19.1	21.5	18.0	23.4	18.9	21.6
6.	Lakshadweep	21.7	28.4	20.9	29.3	19.9	30.2
7.	Pondicherry	16.2	19.2	16.2	19.8	15.3	19.7

N.A. Not available due to part receipt of returns.

Rate				Infant Morrtality Rate						
Rural		Urban		Total		Rural		Urban		India/States/
Lower Limit	Upper Limit	Lower Limit	Upper Limit	Lower Limit	Upper Limit	Lower Limit	Upper Limit	Lower Limit	Upper Limit	Union Territories
10	11	12	13	14	15	16	17	18	19	1
9.3	**9.6**	**6.1**	**6.5**	**68.3**	**71.7**	**73.5**	**77.3**	**40.1**	**47.3**	**India**
										Bigger States
8.5	9.4	5.1	6.3	59.4	72.9	66.9	83.2	27.8	45.6	1. Andhra Pradesh
9.0	11.2	5.3	7.0	67.5	83.7	70.0	87.3	24.7	47.0	2. Assam
8.8	9.6	6.1	8.0	60.4	70.8	61.2	72.3	40.4	62.3	3. Bihar
8.3	9.3	5.1	6.6	56.3	70.0	62.4	77.8	31.1	58.2	4. Gujarat
7.8	9.2	5.6	7.1	60.2	75.1	61.6	78.4	40.7	75.4	5. Haryana
8.3	9.1	4.9	6.2	52.2	64.9	61.8	77.0	14.3	35.5	6. Karnataka
6.1	6.8	5.6	6.9	11.3	17.6	10.9	16.8	7.4	25.4	7. Kerala
10.6	11.7	6.8	8.5	84.3	96.8	88.7	102.3	41.1	69.8	8. Madhya Pradcsh
8.2	9.1	5.1	6.2	42.4	53.9	50.9	65.5	22.5	40.1	9. Maharashtra
10.5	11.7	6.2	8.1	87.3	106.2	89.9	110.6	49.3	79.8	10. Orissa
7.3	8.4	5.4	6.8	45.9	60.4	48.4	65.5	26.2	52.3	11. Punjab
8.3	9.4	5.7	7.1	75.5	86.9	78.5	91.2	47.3	71.0	12. Rajasthan

10	*11*	*12*	*13*	*14*	*15*	*16*	*17*	*18*	*19*	*1*
8.3	9.2	6.0	7.1	46.0	58.2	50.1	65.7	30.2	47.7	13. Tamil Nadu
10.7	11.5	7.4	8.8	79.7	87.8	82.4	91.3	54.4	73.6	14. Uttar Pradesh
6.8	7.5	6.3	7.3	47.4	56.8	49.4	60.0	30.6	49.9	15. West Bengal
										Smaller States
										1. Arunachal Pradesh
										2. Chhatisgarh
										3. Goa
										4. Jharkhand
										5. Himachal Pradcsh
										6. Jammu & Kashmir
										7. Manipur
										8. Meghalaya
										9. Mizoram
										10. Nagaland
										11. Sikkim
										12. Tripura
										13. Uttaranchal
										Union Territories
										1. Andaman & Nicobar Islands

Confidence limits of Death rate Infant Mortality Rate for smaller states and union territories have not been presented due to the small sample size and very large variations between the Upper and Lower tolerance limits.

10	11	12	13	14	15	16	17	18	19	1
										2. Chandigarh
										3. Dadra & Nagar Haveli
										4. Daman & Diu
										5. Delhi
										6. Lakshadweep
										7. Pondicherry

Table 3

India/States/ Union Territories	Total			Rural			Urban		
	Total	Male	Female	Total	Male	Female	Total	Male	Female
1	2	3	4	5	6	7	8	9	10
India	**8.7**	**9.0**	**8.3**	**9.4**	**9.7**	**9.1**	**6.3**	**6.7**	**5.8**
Bigger States									
1. Andhra Pradesh	8.2	9.0	7.4	9.0	9.8	8.1	5.7	6.4	5.0
2. Assam	9.7	10.2	9.2	10.1	10.5	9.6	6.2	6.9	5.3
3. Bihar	8.9	8.4	9.5	9.2	8.7	9.7	7.1	6.7	7.5
4. Gujarat	7.9	8.5	7.2	8.8	9.6	8.0	5.9	6.2	5.6
5. Haryana	7.7	7.7	7.7	8.0	8.0	8.0	6.4	6.4	6.4
6. Karnataka	7.7	S.5	7.0	8.7	9.4	8.0	5.5	6.3	4.7
7. Kerala	6.4	7.5	5.4	6.5	7.7	5.4	6.3	7.0	5.6
8. Madhya Pradesh	10.4	10.6	10.3	11.1	11.3	11.0	7.6	7.9	7.3
9. Maharashtra	7.5	8.2	6.7	8.7	9.3	8.1	5.6	6.6	4.5
10. Orissa	10.7	10.9	10.4	11.1	11.4	10.9	7.1	7.2	7.1
11. Punjab	7.4	8.1	6.7	7.9	8.6	7.0	6.1	6.5	5.7
12. Rajasthan	8.4	8.9	7.9	8.9	9.2	8.5	6.4	7.4	5.4
13. Tamil Nadu	8.0	8.8	7.3	8.7	9.5	8.0	6.6	7.3	5.8

1	2	3	4	5	6	7	8	9	10
14. Uttar Pradesh	10.5	10.4	10.7	11.1	11.0	11.2	8.1	7.8	8.3
15. West Bengal	7.1	7.2	6.9	7.2	7.2	7.1	6.8	7.3	6.3
Smaller States									
1. Arunachal Pradesh	6.0	6.4	5.7	6.4	6.8	6.1	1.9	2.2	1.6
2. Chhatisgarh	9.6	10.7	8.4	11.3	13.1	9.5	7.0	7.4	6.7
3. Goa	7.2	8.4	6.1	7.6	8.7	6.6	6.6	7.9	5.3
4. Jharkhand	8.9	8.8	9.0	9.7	9.4	9.9	6.4	6.9	5.8
5. Himachal Pradesh	7.3	8.2	6.5	7.5	8.5	6.6	5.2	5.6	4.8
7. Jammu & Kashmir	Data notcomplied due to pan receipt of returns								
8. Manipur	5.4	6.4	4.5	5.0	6.1	4.0	6.6	7.3	5.8
9. Meghalaya	9.1	10.2	8.0	10.2	11.5	9.0	3.3	3.7	2.8
10. Mizoram	5.5	7.1	3.9	6.9	8.9	5.0	3.7	5.0	2.5
11. Nagaland	2.3	1.3	3.5	N.A.	N.A.	N.A.	2.3	1.3	3.5
12. Sikkim	5.8	5.4	6.2	5.9	5.5	6.4	3.4	4.5	2.2
13. Tripura	5.7	6.3	5.1	5.7	6.4	4.9	5.7	5.5	5.9
14. Uttaranchal	6.5	6.9	5.9	10.5	11.2	9.7	3.5	3.9	3.1

1	2	3	4	5	6	7	8	9	10
Union Territories									
1. Andaman & Nicobar Islands	5.5	5.8	5.3	6.2	7.0	5.4	3.5	2.2	4.9
2. Chandigarh	3.9	3.7	4.1	2.6	1.7	4.0	4.1	4.0	4.1
3. Dadra & Nagar Haveli	6.6	7.4	5.9	7.0	7.8	6.2	2.5	3.1	1.8
4. Daman & Diu	7.1	7.2	6.9	8.9	9.8	7.9	5.4	4.8	6.1
5. Delhi	4.8	5.3	4.3	4.5	4.7	4.4	4.9	5.3	4.3
6. Lakshadweep	4.7	4.8.	4.5	4.3	4.2	4.4	5.0	5.4	4.6
7. Pondicherry	6.9	8.3	5.4	7.9	9.0	6.8	6.1	7.8	4.5

N.A. Not available due to part receipt of returns.
Note: Estimates of Death rate by sex are subject to year to year fluctuations.

Table 4 : Infant mortality rate by sex, 1999

India/States/ Union Territories	*Total*			*Rural*			*Urban*		
	Total	*Male*	*Female*	*Total*	*Male*	*Female*	*Total*	*Male*	*Female*
1	*2*	*3*	*4*	*5*	*6*	*7*	*8*	*9*	*10*
India	**70.0**	**69.8**	**70.8**	**75.4**	**75.6**	**75.2**	**43.8**	**47.4**	**39.7**
Bigger States									
1. Andhra Pradesh	66.3	68.9	63.5	75.4	79.2	70.6	37.4	35.1	39.9
2. Assam	75.6	74.7	76.4	78.6	77.8	79.5	35.8	36.1	35.6
3. Bihar	62.8	63.2	62.3	63.6	64.3	62.8	55.1	52.5	57.7
4. Gujarat	63.2	61.7	64.8	70.1	67.9	72.6	44.6	45.7	43.3
5. Haryana	67.7	59.1	78.4	69.8	56.8	86.1	58.0	69.4	43.5
6. Karnataka	57.7	58.6	56.7	69.4	73.4	65.1	24.5	18.5	31.5
7. Kerala	14.5	13.7	15.3	13.8	12.4	15.4	16.4	18.0	14.9
8. Madhya Pradesh	89.5	89.6	89.5	95.8	94.9	96.8	55.3	59.6	50.7
9. Maharashtra	48.2	47.8	48.5	58.2	64.1	51.9	31.3	20.5	42.8
10. Orissa	96.7	97.3	96.0	100.2	101.2	99.2	64.6	63.8	65.5
11. Punjab	53.1	50.5	56.4	57.0	48.8	67.2	39.3	56.5	16.2
12. Rajasthan	81.2	78.9	83.9	84.7	79.9	90.5	59.1	73.5	40.5

	1	2	3	4	5	6	7	8	9	10
13.	Tamil Nadu	52.4	50.3	54.5	58.1	57.5	58.8	39.4	33.8	45.1
14.	Uttar Pradesh	84.4	85.2	83.5	87.6	86.1	89.4	65.8	80.1	49.6
15.	West Bengal	52.1	60.7	43.0	54.7	61.9	47:1	40.3	55.1	24.0
Smaller States										
1.	Arunachal Pradesh	35.4	43.0	27.9	37.4	46.0	29.2	N.A.	N.A.	N.A.
2.	Chhatisgarh	77.6	92.1	62.0	94.5	116.5	71.3	47.1	49.4	44.4
3.	Goa	16.7	26.3	6.6	22.3	32.0	11.4	8.5	17.2	0.0
4.	Jharkhand	71.2	63.7	79.1	76.1	69.8	82.6	48.1	34.0	62.4
5.	Himachal Pradesh	54.1	56.9	51.1	55.0	58.0	51.9	37.0	38.8	34.9
6.	Jammu & Kashmir	Data not compiled due to partreceipt of returns								
7.	Manipur	22.8	22.1	23.7	24.6	25.8	23.1	17.1	9.6	25.7
8.	Meghalaya	61.3	66.6	55.6	64.7	71.4	57.6	25.6	22.2	30.3
9.	Mizoram	13.7	18.8	8.9	14.0	23.2	6.2	13.2	12.8	13.6
10.	Nagaland	31.7	21.3	42.5	N.A.	N.A.	N.A.	31.7	21.3	42.5
11.	Sikkim	46.1	49.7	42.4	46.8	50.3	43.3	17.6	29.4	0.0
12.	Tripura	27.1	22.6	31.8	26.9	23.8	30.2	28.5	14.6	40.9
13.	Uttaranchal	52.4	60.0	43.8	75.3	65.4	87.4	27.3	53.6	0.0

1	2	3	4	5	6	7	8	9	10
Union Territories									
1. Andaman & Nicobar Islands	13.9	10.5	17.1	17.1	14.4	19.7	5.5	0.0	10.4
2. Chandigarh	15.6	9.0	23.7	22.5	0.0	58.8	14.5	10.8	18.9
3. Dadra & Nagar Haveli	42.3	57.7	27.0	44.9	61.1	28.7	0.0	0.0	0.0
4. Daman & Diu	6.8	12.0	2.9	15.6	22.1	8.2	0.0	0.0	0.0
5. Delhi	25.4	29.1	20.5	27.8	27.3	28.4	25.1	29.3	19.5
6. Lakshadweep	21.3	29.1	13.8	34.1	55.0	10.4	9.1	0.0	16.7
7. Pondicherry	20.9	31.1	10.2	27.4	32.0	23.2	16.3	30.5	0.0

N.A. Not available due to part receipt of returns.
Note: Estimates of Infant mortality rate by sex are subject to year to year fluctuations.

ABOUT THE SAMPLE REGISTRATION SYSTEM (SRS)

The Sample Registration System (SRS) is a large scale demographic survey for providing reliable annual estimates of birth rate, death rate and other fertility and mortality indicators at the national and sub-national levels. The field investigation consists of continuous enumeration of births and deaths by a resident part time enumerator, generally a teacher and an independent survey, every six months by a departmental official. The data obtained through these operations are matched. The unmatched and partially matched events are re-verified in the field and thereafter an unduplicated count of births and deaths is obtained. The SRS was initiated by the OFFICE OF THE REGISTRAR GENERAL, INDIA on a pilot basis in a few selected states in 1964-65 and it became fully operational during 1969-70 with about 3700 sample units. Thereafter the number of sample units was periodically increased and the frame updated after each census. The latest updating based on the 1991 census data was done in 1993-1994. The sample unit in rural areas is a village or a segment of it if the village had a population of 1500 or more. In urban areas the sampling unit is a census enumeration block with a population ranging from 750 to 1000. At present SRS has 6671 sample units (4436 rural and 2235 urban) in all States and Union territories covering about 1.1 million households and 6.05 million population. The state-wise break up of the sample units and the population covered are given below :

Number of sample units and population covered India, States and Union Territories 1999

India/States/	*Number of sample units*			*Population covered (in '000)*		
Union Territories	*Total*	*Rural*	*Urban*	*Total*	*Rural*	*Urban*
1	*2*	*3*	*4*	*5*	*6*	*7*
India	**6671**	**4436**	**2235**	**6047**	**4725**	**1322**
Bigger States						
1. Andhra Pradesh	310	210	100	306	240	66
2. Assam	275	200	75	238	195	43

1	2	3	4	5	6	7
3. Bihar	361	308	53	428	393	34
4. Gujarat	300	200	100	274	222	51
5. Haryana	180	110	70	209	159	50
6. Karnataka	375	260	115	353	281	72
7. Kerala	250	150	100	302	240	62
8. Madhya Pradesh	299	216	83	292	243	49
9. Maharashtra	375	200	175	337	232	105
10. Orissa	405	300	105	300	239	61
11. Punjab	200	120	80	175	127	48
12. Rajasthan	350	250	100	325	277	48
13. Tamil Nadu	375	200	175	350	234	116
14. Uttar Pradesh	615	428	187	633	531	102
15. West Bengal	475	300	175	465	357	108
Smaller States						
1. Arunachal Pradesh	56	50	6	45	38	7
2. Chhatisgarh	101	84	17	90	80	10
3. Goa	70	40	30	62	44	17
4. Jharkhand	139	92	47	119	94	25

	1	2	3	4	5	6	7
5.	Himachal Pradesh	190	140	50	100	72	28
6.	Jammu & Kashmir	166	100	66	Not available	Not available	Not available
7.	Manipur	150	100	50	132	97	35
8.	Meghalaya	120	100	20	60	51	10
9.	Mizoram	32	16	16	22	12	11
10.	Nagaland	35	25	10	Not available	Not available	5
11.	Sikkim	60	50	10	57	49	9
12.	Tripura	75	60	15	87	78	9
13.	Uttaranchal	35	22	13	30	24	6
Union Territories							
1.	Andaman & Nicobar Islands	45	30	15	31	22	9
2.	Chandigarh	30	5	25	27	7	20
3.	Dadra & Nagar Haveli	25	20	5	26	23	4
4.	Daman & Diu	17	15	2	20	19	1
5.	Delhi	130	10	120	98	16	83
6.	Lakshadweep	10	5	5	13	8	4
7.	Pondicherry	40	20	20	36	22	13

Note: Total population may not add up to the sum of Rural and Urban population due to rounding.

VOLUME 36 NO. 2 OCTOBER 2002

SAMPLE REGISTRATION SYSTEM BULLETIN

PUBLISHED BI-ANNUALLY IN APRIL AND OCTOBER EACH YEAR-ISSN 0971-3549

REGISTRAR GENERAL, INDIA

Vital Statistics Division, West Block 1, Wing 1, 2nd Floor, R.K. Puram, New Delhi-110 066

Table 1. Provisional Estimates of Bith rate, Birth Rate, Natural growth rate and Infant mortality rate, 2001

India / States / Union Territories	*Birth rate*			*Death rate*			*Natural growth rate*			*Infant mortality rate*		
	Total	*Rural*	*Urban*	*Total*	*Rural*	*Urban*	*Total*	*Rural*	*Urban*	*Total*	*Rural*	*Urban*
1	*2*	*3*	*4*	*5*	*6*	*7*	*8*	*9*	*10*	*11*	*12*	*13*
India *25.4	**27.1**	**20.2**	**8.4**	**9.0**	**6.3**	**17.0**	**18.0**	**13.9**	**66**	**72**	**42**	
Bigger States												
1. Andhra Pradesh	20.8	21.3	19.6	8.1	8.9	5.6	12.8	12.4	14.0	66	74	39
2. Assam	26.8	27.8	18.5	9.5	9.8	6.6	17.3	18.0	11.9	73	76	33
3. Bihar	31.2	32.3	23.4	8.2	8.5	6.3	23.0	23.7	17.1	62	63	52
4. Gujarat	24.9	26.6	21.5	7.8	8.8	5.6	17.2	17.8	15.9	60	67	42
5. Haryana	26.7	27.8	22.8	7.6	7.6	7.4	19.1	20.2	15.4	65	68	54
6. Karnataka	22.2	23.6	19.0	7.6	8.2	6.4	14.6	15.4	12.6	58	69	27
7. Kerala	17.2	17.4	16.6	6.6	6.8	6.1	10.6	10.6	10.5	11	12	9

1	2	3	4	5	6	7	8	9	10	11	12	13
8. Madhya Pradesh	30.8	32.8	23.0	10.0	10.8	7 2	20.8	22.0	15.9	86	92	53
9. Maharashtra	20.6	21.0	20.1	7.5	8.5	5.9	13.1	12.5	14.2	45	55	27
10. Orissa	23.4	23.9	19.6	10.2	10.7	6.8	13.1	13.2	12.8	90	94	60
11. Punjab	21.2	22.1	18.7	7.0	7.2	6.4	14.2	14.8	12.2	51	55	37
12. Rajasthan	31.0	32.3	24.7	7.9	8.3	6.2	23.0	24.0	18.5	79	83	57
13. Tamil Nadu	19.0	19.6	17.8	7.6	8.4	6.0	11.4	11.2	11.8	49	54	35
14. Uttar Pradesh	32.1	33.2	27.0	10.1	10.6	7.8	22.0	22.5	19.2	82	86	62
15. West Bengal	20.5	22.8	13.S	6.8	7.0	6.4	13.7	15.8	7.4	51	53	38
Smaller States												
1. Arunachal Pradesh	22.0	22.9	12.8	5.5	5.9	2.3	16.5	17.0	10.6	39	41	11
2. Chhatisgarh	26.3	29.0	22.4	8.8	10.1	7.0	17.5	18.9	15.4	76	88	56
3. Goa	13.9	14.0	13.9	7.5	8.1	6.5	6.5	5.9	7.4	19	21	16
4. Jharkhand	26.3	28.3	19.5	8.8	9.7	6.0	17.4	18.6	13.4	62	67	40
5. Himachal Pradesh	21.0	21.3	16.8	7.0	7.1	5.3	14.0	14.2	11.5	54	55	32
6. Jammu & Kashmir	20.1	21.1	16.3	6.1	6.1	6.0	14.1	15.0	10.3	48	50	39
7. Manipur	18.2	19.0	15.9	5.1	4.8	6.1	13.1	14.2	9.9	20	19	23
8. Meghalaya	28.3	30.7	15.0	9.0	9.9	3.9	19.3	20.7	11.1	56	57	41
9. Mizoram	15.7	17.7	13.2	4.4	5.2	3.4	11.3	12.4	9.8	19	23	12

	1	2	3	4	5	6	7	8	9	10	11	12	13
10.	Nagaland	N.A.	N.A.	12.4	N.A.	N.A.	2.6	N.A.	N.A.	9.9	N.A.	N.A.	13
11.	Sikkim	21.6	21.8	16.7	5.1	5.2	3.2	16.5	16.6	13.5	42	43	31
12.	Tripura	16.1	16.6	13.5	5.6	5.6	5.2	10.5	11.0	8.3	39	40	30
13.	Uttaranchal	18.5	21.1	16.6	7.8	10.0	6.1	10.7	11.1	10.5	48	69	26
Union Territories													
1.	Andaman & Nicobar Islands	16.8	17.8	14.2	4.7	5.0	4.1	12.1	12.8	10.2	18	21	8
2.	Chandigarh	16.1	20.6	15.6	3.5	2.2	3.7	12.6	18.4	11.9	24	28	23
3.	Dadra & Nagar Haveli	29.3	30.1	20.0	6.5	6.8	2.9	22.8	23.3	17.1	58	62	9
4.	Daman & Diu	22.3	22.6	22.0	6.7	7.6	5.9	15.6	15.0	16.2	40	42	35
5.	Delhi	18.7	23.2	18.1	5.0	5.4	5.0	13.6	17.8	13.1	29	34	28
6.	Lakshadweep	20.4	22.1	18.7	5.0	4.7	5.2	15.4	17.4	13.5	33	34	33
7.	Pondicherry	17.9	18.7	17.3	7.0	7.7	6.6	10.8	11.0	10.7	22	31	15

* Excludes Nagaland (Rural) due to part-receipt of returns.
N.A.: Not available due to part-receipt of returns.
Note : Infant mortality rates for Smaller States and Union Territories are for the period 1999-2001.

With compliments from Jayant Kumar Banthia, Registrar General, India, 2-A Mansingh Road, New Delhi-110 011, India.
E-mail : orgindia @vsnl.net Phone : ((91) (11) 338 3761 Fax : (91) (11) 338 3145
Census and Vital Statistics Website on the Internet : http://www.censusindia.net.

Table 2. Estimates of birth rate, death rate and infant mortality rate for the latest three years, 1998-2000

India / States / Union Territories	*Year*	*Birth rate*			*Death rate*			*Infant mortality rate*		
		Total	*Rural*	*Urban*	*Total*	*Rural*	*Urban*	*Total*	*Rural*	*Urban*
1	*2*	*3*	*4*	*5*	*6*	*7*	*8*	*9*	*10*	*11*
India *1998	**26.5**	**28.0**	**21.1**	**9.0**	**9.7**	**6.6**	**72**	**77**	**45**	
	1999	**26.0**	**27.6**	**20.8**	**8.7**	**9.4**	**6.3**	**70**	**75**	**44**
	2000	**25.8**	**27.6**	**20.7**	**8.5**	**9.3**	**6.3**	**68**	**74**	**44**
Bigger States										
1. Andhra Pradesh	1998	22.4	22.8	21.1	8.8	9.7	6.1	66	75	38
	1999	21.7	22.0	20.6	8.2	9.0	5.7	66	75	37
	2000	21.3	21.7	20.1	8.2	9.0	5.8	65	74	36
2. Assam	1998	27.9	28.7	20.2	10.0	10.5	6.0	76	80	36
	1999	27.0	28.0	18.9	9.7	10.1	6.2	76	79	36
	2000	26.9	27.9	18.6	9.6	10.0	6.1	75	78	35
3. Bihar	1998	31.1	32.1	23.1	9.4	9.7	6.5	67	68	51
	1999	31.5	32.4	25.2	8.9	9.2	7.1	63	64	55
	2000	31.9	32.8	25.6	8.8	9.1	7.1	62	63	53
4. Gujarat	1998	25.5	27.0	22.2	7.9	8.6	6.4	64	71	46

1	2	3	4	5	6	7	8	9	10	11
	1999	25.4	27.0	22.0	7.9	8.8	5..9	63	70	45
	2000	25.2	26.8	21.9	7.5	8.3	5.8	62	69	45
5. Haryana	1998	27.6	28.8	23.3	8.2	8.6	6.9	70	72	59
	1999	26.8	27.7	23.3	7.7	8.0	6.4	68	70	58
	2000	26.9	28.0	23.1	7.5	7.9	6.2	67	69	57
6. Karnataka	1998	22.0	23.1	19.4	7.9	8.9	5.6	58	70	25
	1999	22.3	23.7	19.2	7.7	8.7	5.5	58	69	24
	2000	22.0	23.3	19.1	7.8	S.6	5.8	57	68	24
7. Kerala	1998	18.3	18.3	18.2	6.4	6.5	6.2	16	15	17
	1999	18.0	18.1	17.7	6.4	6.5	6.3	14	14	16
	2000	17.9	18.0	17.5	6.4	6.5	6.2	14	14	14
8. Madhya Pradesh	1998	30.7	32.1	23.1	11.2	11.9	7.8	98	104	56
	1999	31.1	33.1	23.6	10.4	11. 1	7.6	90	96	55
	2000	31.4	33.4	23.5	10.3	11.1	7.5	87	93	54
9. Maharashtra	1998	22.5	23.6	20.8	7.7	8.9	5.8	49	58	32
	1999	21.1	21.6	20.3	7.5	8.7	5.6	48	58	31
	2000	21.0	21.4	20.4	7.5	8.6	5.8	48	56	33

1		2	3	4	5	6	7	8	9	10	11
10.	Orissa	1998	25.7	26.4	20.9	11.1	11.6	7.6	98	101	66
		1999	24.1	24.6	20.3	10.7	11.1	7.1	97	100	65
		2000	24.3	24.9	20.1	10.5	11.0	7.0	95	99	66
11.	Punjab	1998	22.4	23.7	18.5	7.7	8.2	6.3	54	58	40
		1999	21.5	22.5	18.6	7.4	7.9	6.1	53	57	39
		2000	21.6	20.7	18.6	7.4	7.9	5.9	52	56	38
12.	Rajasthan	1998	31.6	33.1	247	8.8	9.3	6.9	83	87	60
		1999	31.1	32.5	24.9	8.4	8.9	6.4	81	85	59
		2000	31.4	32.8	25.1	8.5	8.9	6.6	79	82	58
13.	Tamil Nadu	1998	19.2	19.7	18.1	8.5	9.3	6.8	53	59	40
		1999	19.3	19.8	18.2	8.0	8.7	6.6	52	58	39
		2000	19.3	20.0	18.1	7.9	8.7	6.5	51	56	38
14.	Uttar Pradesh	1998	32.4	33.4	27.2	10.5	10.9	8.1	85	89	65
		1999	32.8	33.9	27.5	10.5	11.1	8.1	84	88	66
		2000	32.8	34.0	27.2	10.3	10.8	8.0	83	87	65
15.	West Bengal	1998	21.3	23.4	15.2	7.5	7.7	7.1	53	56	41
		1999	20.7	22.9	14.3	7.1	7.2	6.S	52	55	40
		2000	20.7	23.0	14.1	7.0	7.2	6.7	51	54	37

1	2	3	4	5	6	7	8	9	10	11
Smaller States										
1. Arunachal Pradesh	1998	22.5	23.3	13.6	6.1	6.5	1.8	44	46	10
	1999	22.3	23.2	13.5	6.0	6.4	1.9	43	45	10
	2000	22.3	23.1	13.9	6.0	6.3	2.5	44	45	11
2. Chhatisgarh	1998	Included in Madhya Pradesh								
	1999	26.9	29.3	23.6	9.6	11.3	7.0	78	95	47
	2000	26.7	29.2	22.8	9.6	11.2	7.1	79	95	49
3. Goa	1998	14.3	14.6	14.0	S.2	8.5	7.9	23	25	22
	1999	14.3	14.4	14.1	7.2	7.6	6.6	21	23	17
	2000	14.3	14.3	14.2	7.4	7.9	6.7	23	24	21
4. Jharkhand	1998	Included in Bihar								
	1999	26.3	28.5	19.0	8.9	9.7	6.4	71	76	48
	2000	26.5	28.8	19.4	9.0	9.8	6.5	70	74	48
5. Himachal Pradesh	1998	22.6	23.0	17.0	7.7	7.9	5.4	64	66	38
	1999	23.8	24.3	16.8	7.3	7.5	5.2	62	63	38
	2000	22.1	22.5	16.9	7.2	7.3	5.5	60	62	37
6. Jammu & Kashmir	1998	19.9	20.8	16.1	5.4	5.6	4.6	45	46	44
	1999	20.9	22.0	16.5	6.3	6.2	6.3	52	53	44
	2000	19.7	20.5	16.5	6.2	6.3	5.9	50	51	45

1		*2*	*3*	*4*	*5*	*6*	*7*	*8*	*9*	*10*	*11*
7.	Manipur	1998	19.0	19.9	16.7	5.3	5.1	6.1	25	22	26
		1999	18.6	19.4	16.4	5.4	5.0	6.6	25	22	24
		2000	18.3	19.1	16.2	5.6	5.4	6.0	23	23	25
8.	Meghalaya	1998	29.2	31.8	15.6	9.0	9.9	4.2	52	54	36
		1999	28.7	31.1	15.7	9.1	10.2	3.3	56	59	33
		2000	28.5	31.0	15.3	9.2	10.1	4.6	58	61	32
9.	Mizoram	1998	15.8	18.1	13.1	5.6	6.7	4.3	23	26	18
		1999	17.0	18.7	14.8	5.5	6.9	3.7	19	22	14
		2000	16.0	19.2	12.2	5.2	6.2	3.9	21	23	17
10.	Nagaland	1998	N.A	N.A	11.9	N.A	N.A	1.7	N,A	N.A	16
		1999	N.A	N.A	11.8	N.A	N.A	2.3	N.A	N.A	16
		2000	N.A	N.A	12.2	N.A	N.A	3.0	N.A	N.A	23
11.	Sikkim	1998	20.9	21.2	13.5	6.1	6.2	3.9	52	52	44
		1999	21.6	21.9	14.7	5.8	5.9	3.4	49	50	33
		2000	21.8	22.1	14.8	5.7	5.7	4.0	49	49	36
12.	Tripura	1998	17.6	18.2	14.8	6.1	6.2	5.4	49	50	39
		1999	17.0	17.5	14.4	5.7	5.7	5.7	42	43	33
		2000	16.5	17.0	14.0	5.4	5.3	5.6	41	42	32

1		2	3	4	5	6	7	8	9	10	11
13.	Uttaranchal	1998	Included in Uttar Pradesh								
		1999	19.6	24.5	16.1	6.5	10.5	3.5	52	75	27
		2000	20.2	24.6	17.1	6.9	10.3	4.5	50	73	26
Union Territories											
1.	Andaman & Nicobar Islands	1998	17.7	18.0	16.8	4.6	5.1	3.0	30	37	9
		1999	18.1	17.8	19.2	5.5	6.2	3.5	25	30	9
		2000	19.1	19.0	19-3	5.1	5.7	3.4	23	27	10
2.	Chandigarh	1998	17.9	21.3	17.5	4.1	3.5	4.2	32	44	30
		1999	17.9	24.5	17.1	3.9	2.6	4.1	28	36	27
		2000	17.5	18.9	17.3	3.9	3.8	3.9	28	38	26
3.	Dadra & Nagar Haveli	1998	34.1	35.1	23.4	7.9	8.4	3.0	61	65	7
		1999	34.2	35.2	23.6	6.6	7.0	2.5	56	61	7
		2000	34.9	35.9	24.0	7.8	8.2	3.5	58	62	14
4.	Daman & Diu	1998	21.7	23.0	20.5	7.0	8.1	6.1	51	42	59
		1999	26.9	24.9	28.8	7.1	8.9	5.4	35	34	36
		2000	23.7	21.8	25.4	6.6	7.1	6.2	48	38	57

1		2	3	4	5	6	7	8	9	10	11
5.	Delhi	1998	19.4	20.9	19.3	5.3	5.3	5.3	36	36	36
		1999	20.3	20.7	20.3	4.8	4.5	4.9	31	33	31
		2000	20.3	21.4	20.1	5.1	5.0	s.r	32	32	32
6.	Lakshadweep	1998	23.0	23.5	22.4	6.2	6.1	6.2	26	22	30
		1999	25.1	25.1	25.0	4.7	4.3	5.0	32	26	37
		2000	26.1	27.6	24.6	6.0	7.1	4.9	27	25	29
7.	Pondicherry	1998	18.2	18.3	18.1	7.8	8.7	7.2	21	31	14
		1999	17.7	18.0	17.5	6.9	7.9	6.1	22	32	15
		2000	17.8	18.4	17.4	6.5	7.2	6.0	23	33	15

* Excludes Nagaland (Rural) due to part-receipt of returns.

N.A. Not available due to non-receipt of returns.

Note: Infant mortality rate for smaller states/Ut's shown against 1998, 1999 and 2000 are for the periods 1996-98, 1997-99 and 1998-2000 respectively.

About the Sample Registration System (SRS)

The Sample Registration System (SRS) is a large scale demographic survey for providing reliable annual estimates of birth rate, death rate and other fertility and mortality indicators at the national and sub-national levels. The vital rates in respect of the three newly created states of Chhatisgarh, Jharkhand and Uttaranchal were first published for the year 1999 in the April, 2001 issue of SRS bulletin and were continued for subsequent years. The present issue also contains the vital rates for 2001 for these states. The field investigation consists of continuous enumeration of births and deaths by a resident_part time enumerator, generally a teacher and an independent survey every six months by a computer supervisor. The data obtained through these operations are matched. The unmatched and partially matched events are re-verified in the field and thereafter an unduplicated count of births and deaths is obtained. The SRS was initiated by the OFFICE OF THE REGISTRAR GENERAL, INDIA on a pilot basis in a few selected states in 1964-65 and it became fully operational during 1969-70 with about 3700 sample units. Thereafter the number of sample units was periodically increased. The sample unit in rural areas is a village or a segment of it if the village had a population of 1500 or more. In urban areas the sampling unit is a census enumeration block with a population ranging from 750 to 1000. At present SRS has 6671 sample units (4436 rural and 2235 urban) in all States and Union territories covering about 1.1 million households and 6.33 million population.

VOLUME 37 NO. 2 OCTOBER 2003

SAMPLE REGISTRATION SYSTEM BULLETIN

PUBLISHED BI-ANNUALLY IN APRIL AND OCTOBER EACH YEAR-ISSN 0971-3549

REGISTRAR GENERAL, INDIA

Vital Statistics Division, West Block 1, Wing 1, 2nd Floor, R.K. Puram, New Delhi-110 066

Table 1. Provisional Estimates of Bith rate, Birth rate, Natural growth rate and Infant mortality rate, 2002

India / States / Union Territories	*Birth rate*			*Death rate*			*Natural growth rate*			*Infant mortality rate*		
	Total	*Rural*	*Urban*	*Total*	*Rural*	*Urban*	*Total*	*Rural*	*Urban*	*Total*	*Rural*	*Urban*
1	*2*	*3*	*4*	*5*	*6*	*7*	*8*	*9*	*10*	*11*	*12*	*13*
India *25.0	**26.6**	**19.9**	**8.1**	**8.7**	**6.1**	**16.9**	**17.9**	**13.9**	**64**	**69**	**40**	
Bigger States												
1. Andhra Pradesh	20.6	21.0	19.2	8.0	8.8	5.4	12.6	12.2	13.7	62	71	35
2. Assam	26.6	27.5	18.3	9.2	9.6	6.0	17.4	18.0	12.3	70	73	38
3. Bihar	30.9	31.8	23.5	7.9	8.2	6.1	23.0	23.7	17.4	61	62	50
4. Gujarat	24.6	26.5	20.5	7.6	8.3	6.3	17.0	18.3	14.2	60	68	37
5. Haryana	26.5	27.5	22.5	7.0	7.2	6.3	19.5	20.4	16.2	62	65	51
6. Karnataka	22.0	23.4	18.8	7.2	7.8	5.7	14.9	15.6	13.0	55	65	25
7. Kerala	16.8	17.0	16.3	6.4	6.4	6.2	10.5	10.6	10.2	10	11	8

1	2	3	4	5	6	7	8	9	10	11	12	13
8. Madhya Pradesh	30.3	32.2	22.7	9.7	10.4	7.2	20.6	21.8	15.4	85	90	56
9. Maharashtra	20.2	20.5	19.8	7,3	8.3	5.6	12.9	12.2	14.1	45	52	34
10. Orissa	23.1	23.6	19.5	9.8	10.3	6.3	13.3	13.3	13.2	87	91	56
11. Punjab	20.8	21.7	18.1	7.1	7.4	6.2	13.7	14.4	11.8	51	55	35
12. Rajasthan	30.6	31.9	24.2	7.7	8.0	6.4	22.9	24.0	17.8	78	81	55
13. Tamil Nadu	18.5	19.1	17.5	7.7	8.6	5.9	10.8	10.5	11.5	44	50	32
14. Uttar Pradesh	31.6	32.6	26.8	9.7	10.2	7.3	21.9	22.4	19.5	80	83	58
15. West Bengal	20.3	22.5	14.0	6.6	6.8	6.3	13.7	15.7	7.7	49	52	36
Smaller States												
1. Arunachal Pradesh	20.2	20.9	12.3	4.8	5.0	2.6	15.4	15.9	9.7	40	42	11
2. Chhatisgarh	25.0	26.5	22.6	8.7	9.7	7.2	16.3	16.8	15.4	73	85	51
3. Goa	14.0	14.4	13.5	8.3	9.0	7.2	5.7	5.4	6.3	19	21	16
4. Jharkhand	26.4	28.5	19.0	7.9	8.6	5.8	18.4	20.0	13.1	58	61	38
5. Himachal Pradesh	20.7	21.1	16.5	7.5	7.7	5.1	13.2	13.3	11.4	58	60	32
6. Jammu & Kashmir	19.2	19.9	16.0	5.7	5.7	5.7	13.4	14.1	10.3	47	49	38
7. Manipur	16.8	17.4	15.3	4.6	4.2	5.8	12.2	13.2	9.5	17	17	21
8. Meghalaya	25.8	27.8	14.6	7.7	8.4	3.9	18.1	19.4	10.7	60	62	41
9. Mizoram	16.9	20.8	12.0	4.8	5.7	3.7	12.1	15.1	8.3	15	16	14

1		2	3	4	5	6	7	8	9	10	11	12	13
10.	Nagaland	NA	NA	11.9	NA	NA	2.5	NA	NA	9.4	NA	NA	16
11.	Sikkim	21.9	22.2	13.4	4.9	5.0	4.1	17.0	17.3	9.4	39	39	27
12.	Tripura	14.9	15.3	13.3	5.7	5.6	6.2	9.2	9.6	7.0	38	38	34
13.	Uttaranchal	17.0	18.1	16.2	6.4	9.0	4.4	10.6	9.0	11.8	44	66	22
Union Territories													
1.	Andaman & Nicobar Islands	16.8	17.6	14.6	5.5	6.1	3.8	11.3	11.5	10.7	21	25	8
2.	Chandigarh	14.6	21.5	13.8	3.4	4.1	3.4	11.2	17.4	10.4	25	30	24
3.	Dadra & Nagar Haveli	30.4	31.3	20.4	6.8	7.1	4.0	23.6	24.2	16.3	56	59	16
4.	Daman & Diu	72.4	23.5	21.4	6.6	7.4	5.9	15.8	16.2	15.5	39	35	42
5.	Delhi	17.2	18.2	17.1	5.1	5.7	5.1	12.1	12.4	12.1	32	31	32
6.	Lakshadweep	19.3	20.2	18.3	5.2	5.3	5.1	14.0	14.9	13.2	25	25	25
7.	Pondicherry	17.9	18.1	17.7	6.7	8.1	5.7	11.2	10.1	12.0	23	32	17

* Excludes Nagaland (Rural) due to part-receipt of returns.
N.A.: Not available due to part-receipt of returns.
Note : Infant mortality rates for Smaller States and Union Territories are for the period 2000-2002.

With compliments from Jayant Kumar Banthia, Registrar General, India, 2-A Mansingh Road, New Delhi-110 011, India.
E-mail : orgindia @vsnl.net Phone : ((91) (11) 338 3761 Fax : (91) (11) 338 3145.
Census and Vital Statistics Website on the Internet : http://www.censusindia.net.

Table 2. Estimates of birth rate, death rate and infant mortality rate for the latest three years, 1999-2001

India / States / Union Territories	*Year*	*Birth rate*			*Death rate*			*Infant mortality rate*		
		Total	*Rural*	*Urban*	*Total*	*Rural*	*Urban*	*Total*	*Rural*	*Urban*
1	*2*	*3*	*4*	*5*	*6*	*7*	*8*	*9*	*10*	*11*
India *1999	26.0	27.6	20.8	8.7	9.4	6.3	70	75	44	
	2000	25.8	27.6	20.7	8.5	9.3	6.3	68	74	44
	2001	25.4	27.1	20.3	8.4	9.1	6.3	66	72	42
Bigger States										
1. Andhra Pradesh	1999	21.7	22.0	20.6	8.2	9.0	5.7	66	75	37
	2000	21.3	21.7	20.1	8.2	9.0	5.8	65	74	36
	2001	21.0	21.4	19.7	8.2	9.0	5.6	66	74	40
2. Assam	1999	27.0	28.0	18.9	9.7	10.1	6.2	76	79	36
	2000	26.9	27.9	18.6	9.6	10.0	6.1	75	78	35
	2001	27.0	27.9	18.6	9.6	9.9	6.6	74	77	34
3. Bihar	1999	31.5	32.4	25.2	8.9	9.2	7.1	63	64	55
	2000	31.9	32.8	25.6	8.8	9.1	7.1	62	63	53
	2001	31.2	32.3	23.4	8.2	8.5	6.3	62	63	52

1		*2*	*3*	*4*	*5*	*6*	*7*	*8*	*9*	*10*	*11*
4.	Gujarat	1999	25.4	27.0	22.0	7.9	8.8	5.9	63	70	45
		2000	25.2	26.8	21.9	7.5	8.3	5.8	62	69	45
		2001	25.0	26.7	21.5	7.8	8.9	5.6	60	68	42
5.	Haryana	1999	26.8	27.7	23.3	7.7	8.0	6.4	68	70	58
		2000	26.9	28.0	23.1	7.5	7.9	6.2	67	69	57
		2001	26.8	27.9	22.9	7.6	7.7	7.4	66	68	55
6.	Karnataka	1999	22.3	23.7	19.2	7.7	8.7	5.5	58	69	24
		2000	22.0	23.3	19.1	7.8	8.6	5.8	57	68	24
		2001	22.2	23.6	19.0	7.6	8.2	6.4	58	69	*26*
7.	Kerala	1999	18.0	18.1	17.7	6.4	6.5	6.3	14	14	16
		2000	17.9	18.0	17.5	6.4	6.5	6.2	14	14	14
		2001	17.3	17.4	16.7	6.6	6.8	6.2	11	12	9
8.	Madhya Pradesh	1999	31.1	33.1	23.6	10.4	11.1	7,6	90	96	55
		2000	31.4	33.4	23.5	10.3	11.1	7.5	87	93	54
		2001	31.0	32.9	23.1	10.1	10.8	7.2	86	92	53
9.	Maharashtra	1999	21.1	21.6	20.3	7.5	8.7	5.6	48	58	31
		2000	21.0	21.4	20.4	7.5	8.6	5.8	48	56	33
		2001	20.7	21.1	20.2	7.5	8.5	5.9	45	55	28

1		2	3	4	5	6	7	8	9	10	11
10.	Orissa	1999	24.1	24.6	20.3	10.7	11.1	7.1	97	100	65
		2000	24.3	24.9	20.1	10.5	11.0	7.0	95	99	66
		2001	23.5	24.0	19.7	10.4	10.8	6.8	91	94	61
11.	Punjab	1999	21.5	22.5	18.6	7.4	7.9	6.1	53	57	39
		2000	21.6	22.7	18.6	7.4	7.9	5.9	52	56	38
		2001	21.2	22.1	18.7	7.0	7.2	6.4	52	55	37
12.	Rajasthan	1999	31.1	32.5	24.9	8.4	8.9	6.4	81	85	59
		2000	31.4	32.8	25.1	8.5	8.9	6.6	79	82	58
		2001	31.1	32.4	24.8	8.0	8.3	6.2	80	84	57
13.	Tamil Nadu	1999	19.3	19.8	18.2	8.0	8.7	6.6	52	58	39
		2000	19.3	20.0	18.1	7.9	8.7	6.5	51	56	38
		2001	19.1	19.6	17.8	7.7	8.5	6.0	49	55	35
14.	Uttar Pradesh	1999	32.8	3j.9	27.5	10.5	11.1	8.1	84	88	66
		2000	32.8	34.0	27.2	10.3	10.8	8.0	83	37	65
		2001	32.1	33.2	27.0	10.1	10.6	7.8	83	86	62
15.	West Bengal	1999	20.7	22.9	14.3	7.1	7.2	6.8	52	55	40
		2000	20.7	23.0	14.1	7.0	7.2	6.7	51	54	37
		2001	20.6	22.9	13.8	7.0	7.2	6.4	51	54	37

1		*2*	*3*	*4*	*5*	*6*	*7*	*8*	*9*	*10*	*11*
Smaller States											
1.	Arunachal Pradesh	1999	22.3	23.2	13.5	6.0	6.4	1.9	43	45	10
		2000	22.3	23.1	13.9	6.0	6.3	2.5	4-4	45	11
		2001	22.2	23.1	13.0	5.7	6.0	2.3	39	41	11
2.	Chhatisgarh	1999	26.9	29.3	23.6	9.6	11.3	7.0	78	95	47
		2000	26.7	29.2	22.8	9.6	11.2	7.1	79	95	49
		2001	26.5	29.1	22.5	8.8	10.1	7.0	77	88	58
3.	Goa	1999	14.3	14.4	14.1	7.2	7.6	6.6	21	23	17
		2000	14.3	14.3	14.2	7.4	7.9	6.7	23	24	21
		2001	14.2	14.2	14.2	7.7	8.3	6.7	19	20	15
4.	Jharkhand	1999	26.3	28.5	19.0	8.9	9.7	6.4	71	76	48
		2000	26.5	28.8	19.4	9.0	9.8	6.5	70	74	48
		2001	26.2	2S.3	19.5	8.8	9.7	6.0	62	67	40
5.	HimachaJ Pradesh	1999	23.8	24.3	16.8	7.3	7.5	5.2	62	63	38
		2000	22.1	22.5	16.9,	7.2	7.3	5.5	60	62	37
		2001	21.2	21.5	17.1	7.1	7.2	5.3	54	56	32
6.	Jammu & Kashmir	1999	20.9	22.0	16.5	6.3	6.2	6.3	52	53	44
		2000	19.7	20.5	16.5	6.2	6.3	5.9	50	51	45
		2001	20.2	21.1	16.4	6.1	6.1	6.1	48	49	39

1	2	3	4	5	6	7	8	9	10	11
7. Manipur	1999	18.6	19.4	16.4	5.4	5.0	6.6	25	22	24
	2000	18.3	19.1	16.2	5.6	5.4	6.0	?3	23	25
	2001	18.3	19.0	16.1	5.2	4.8	6.1	20	19	23
8. Meghalaya	1999	28.7	31.1	15.7	9.1	10.2	3.3	56	59	33
	2000	28.5	31.0	15.3	9.2	10.1	4.6	58	61	32
	2001	28.3	30.7	15.0	9.0	9.9	3.9	56	57	41
9. Mizoram	1999	17.0	18.7	14.8	5.5	6.9	3.7	19	22	14
	2000	16.0	19.2	12.2	5.2	6.2	3.9	21	23	17
	2001	15.7	17.7	13.2	4.4	5.2	3.4	19	23	12
10. Nagaland	1999	NA	NA	11.8	NA	NA	2.3	NA	NA	16
	2000	NA	NA	12.2	NA	NA	3.0	NA	NA	23
	2001	NA	NA	12.4	NA	NA	2.6	NA	NA	13
11. Sikkim	1999	21.6	11.9	14.7	5.8	5.9	3.4	49	50	33
	2000	21.8	22.1	14.8	5.7	5.7	4.0	49	49	36
	2001	21.6	21.8	16.7	5.1	5.2	3.2	42	43	31
12. Tripura	1999	17.0	17.5	14.4	5.7	5.7	5.7	42	43	33
	2000	16.5	17.0	14.0	5.4	5.3	5.6	41	42	32
	2001	16.1	16.6	13.5	5.6	5.6	5.2	39	40	30

1		2	3	4	5	6	7	8	9	10	11
13.	Uttaranchal	1999	19.6	24.5	16.1	6.5	10.5	3.5	52	75	27
		2000	20.2	24.6	17.1	6.9	10.3	4.5	50	73	26
		2001	18.5	21.1	16.6	7.8	10.0	6.1.	48	69	26
Union territories											
1.	Andaman & Nicobar Islands	1999	18.1	17.8	19.2	5.5	6.2	3.5	25	30	9
		2000	19.1	19.0	19.3	5.1	5.7	3.4	23	27	10
		2001	16.8	17.8	14.2	4.7	5.0	4.1	18	21	8
2.	Chandigarh	1999	17.9	24.5	17.1	3.9	2.6	4.1	28	36	27
		2000	17.5	18.9	173	3.9	3.8	3.9	28	38	26
		2001	16.3	20.8	15.7	3.6	2.2	3.7	24	28	23
3.	Dadra & Nagar Haveli	1999	34.2	35.2	23.6	6.6	7.0	2.5	56	61	7
		2000	34.9	35.9	24.0	7.8	8.2	3.5	58	62	14
		2001	29.5	30.4	20.0	6.5	6.9	2.9	58	62	9
4.	Daman & Diu	1999	26.9	24.9	28.8	7.1	8.9	5.4	35	34	36
		2000	23.7	21.8	25.4	6.6	7.1	6.2	48	38	57
		2001	22.3	22.7	22.0	6.7	7.6	5.9	40	42	35
5.	Delhi	1999	20.3	20.7	20.3	4.8	4.5	4.9	31	33	31
		2000	20.3	21.4	20.1	5.1	5.0	5.1	32	32	32
		2001	18.9	23.3	18.3	‘5.1	5.6	5.0	29	34	28

1		2	3	4	5	6	7	8	9	10	11
6.	Lakshadweep	1999	25.1	25.1	25.0	4.7	4.3	5.0	32	26	37
		2000	26.1	27.6	24.6	6.0	7.1	4.9	27	25	29
		2001	20.4	22.1	18.7	5.0	4.7	5.2	33	34	33
7.	Pondicherry	1999	17.7	18.0	17.5	6.9	7.9	6.1	22	32	15
		2000	17.8	18.4	17.4	6.5	7.2	6.0	23	33	15
		2001	17.9	18.8	17.3	7.0	7.8	6.6	22	31	15

* Excludes Nagaland (Rural) due to part-receipt of returns.
NA Not available due to part-receipt of returns.
Note: Infant mortality rate for smaller states/UT's shown against 1998, 1999 and 2000 are for the periods 1996-98, 1997-99 and 1998-2000 respectively.

About the Sample Registration System (SRS)

The Sample Registration System (SRS) is a large scale demographic survey for providing reliable annual estimates of birth rate, death rate and other fertility and mortality indicators at the national and sub-national levels. The vital rates in respect of the three newly created states of Chhatisgarh, Jharkhand and Uttaranchal were first published for the year 1999 in the April, 2001 issue of SRS bulletin and were continued for subsequent years. The present issue also contains the vital rates for 2001 for these states. The field investigation consists of continuous enumeration of births and deaths by a resident part time enumerator, generally a teacher and an independent survey every six months by a computer supervisor. The data obtained through these operations are matched. The unmatched and partially matched events are re-verified in the field and thereafter an unduplicated count of births and deaths is obtained. The SRS was initiated by the OFFICE OF THE REGISTRAR GENERAL, INDIA on a pilot basis in a few selected states in 1964-65 and it became fully operational during 1969-70 with about 3700 sample units. Thereafter the number of sample units was periodically increased. The sample unit in rural areas is a village or a segment of it if the village had a population of 1500 or more. In urban areas the sampling unit is a census enumeration block with a population ranging from 750 to 1000. At present SRS has 6671 sample units (4436 rural and 2235 urban) in all States and Union territories covering about 1.1 million households and 6.33 million population.

SRS BULLETIN
SAMPLE REGISTRATION SYSTEM
REGISTRAR GENERAL, INDIA
Vital Statistics Division, West Block 1, Wing 1, 2nd Floor, R.K. Puram, New Delhi-110 066

Table 1. Provisional estimates of Birth rate, Death Rate, Natural growth rate and Infant mortality rate, 2002

India / States / Union Territories	*Birth rate*			*Death rate*			*Natural growth rate*			*Infant mortality rate*		
	Total	*Rural*	*Urban*	*Total*	*Rural*	*Urban*	*Total*	*Rural*	*Urban*	*Total*	*Rural*	*Urban*
1	*2*	*3*	*4*	*5*	*6*	*7*	*8*	*9*	*10*	*11*	*12*	*13*
India*	25.0	26.6	20.0	8.1	8.7	6.1	16.9	17.9	13.9	63	69	40
Bigger States												
1. Andhra Pradesh	20.7	21.1	19.3	8.1	8.9	5.5	12.6	12.2	13.8	62	71	35
2. Assam	26.6	27.5	18.3	9.2	9.6	6.0	17.4	17.9	12.3	70	73	38
3. Bihar	30.9	31.8	23.5	7.9	8.2	6.1	23.0	23.6	17.4	61	62	50
4. Gujarat	24.7	26.6	20.6	7.7	8.3	6.4	17.0	18.3	14.2	60	68	37
5. Haryana	26.6	27.6	22.6	7.1	7.2	6.4	19.5	20.4	16.2	62	64	51
6. Karnataka	22.1	23.5	18.8	7.2	7.9	5.7	14.9	15.6	13.1	55	65	25
7. Kerala	16.9	17.0	16.4	6.4	6.4	6.2	10.5	10.6	10.2	10	11	8

	1	2	3	4	5	6	7	8	9	10	11	12	13
8.	Madhya Pradesh	30.4	32.3	22.7	9.8	10.5	7.2	20.6	21.8	15.5	85	89	56
9.	Maharashtra	20.3	20.6	19.8	7.3	8.3	5.6	13.0	12.3	14.2	45	52	34
10.	Orissa	23.2	23.7	19.6	9.8	10.3	6.4	13.4	13.4	13.2	87	90	56
11.	Punjab	20.8	21.7	18.1	7.1	7.4	6.2	13.7	14.3	11.9	51	55	35
12.	Rajasthan	30.6	31.9	24.2	7.7	8.0	6.4	22.9	23.9	17.8	78	81	55
13.	Tamil Nadu	18.5	19.1	17.5	7.7	8.6	5.9	10.8	10.5	11.6	44	50	32
14.	Uttar Pradesh	31.6	32.6	26.8	9.7	10.2	7.3	21.9	22.4	19.5	80	83	58
15.	West Bengal	20.5	22.6	14.1	6.7	6.9	6.4	13.8	15.7	7.7	49	52	36
Smaller States													
1.	Arunachal Pradesh	20.2	20.9	12.3	4.8	5.0	2.6	15.4	15.9	9.7	37	38	12
2.	Chhatisgarh	25.0	26.5	22.6	8.7	9.7	7.2	16.3	16.8	15.4	73	80	59
3.	Goa	14.0	14.4	13.5	8.3	9.0	7.2	5.7	5.4	6.3	17	19	14
4.	Jharkhand	26.4	28.5	19.0	7.9	8.6	5.8	18.5	19.9	13.2	51	55	33
5.	Himachal Pradesh	20.7	21.1	16.5	7.5	7.7	5.1	13.2	13.4	11.4	52	53	28
6.	Jammu & Kashmir	19.2	19.9	16.0	5.7	5.7	5.7	13.5	14.2	10.3	45	47	34
7.	Manipur	16.8	17.4	15.3	4.6	4.2	5.8	12.2	13.2	9.5	14	12	21
8.	Meghalaya	25.8	27.8	14.6	7.7	8.4	3.9	18.1	19.4	10.7	61	62	49
9.	Mizoram	16.9	20.8	12.0	4.8	5.7	3.7	12.1	15.1	8.3	14	14	14

1		2	3	4	5	6	7	8	9	10	11	12	13
10.	Nagaland	N.A	N.A	11.9	N.A	N.A	2.5	N.A	N.A	9.4	N.A	N.A	15
11.	Sikkim	21.9	22.2	13.4	4.9	5.0	4.1	17.0	17.2	9.3	34	34	25
12.	Tripura	14.9	15.3	13.3	5.7	5.6	6.2	9.2	9.7	7.1	34	35	32
13.	Uttaranchal	17.0	18.1	16.2	6.4	9.0	4.4	10.6	9.1	11.8	41	62	21
Union Territories													
1.	Andaman & Nicobar Islands	16.8	17.6	14.6	5.5	6.1	3.8	11.3	11.5	10.8	15	17	10
2.	Chandigarh	14.6	21.5	13.8	3.4	4.1	3.4	11.2	17.4	10.4	21	25	21
3.	Dadra & Nagar Haveli	30.4	31.3	20.4	6.8	7.1	4.0	23.6	24.2	16.4	56	58	21
4.	Daman & Diu	22.4	23.5	21.4	6.6	7.4	5.9	15.8	16.1	15.5	42	42	43
5.	Delhi	17.2	18.2	17.1	5.1	5.7	5.T	12.1	12.5	12.0	30	31	30
6.	Lakshadweep	19.3	20.2	18.3	5.2	5.3	5.1	14.1	14.9	13.2	25	31	18
7.	Pondicherry	17.9	18.1	17.7	6.7	8.1	5.7	11.2	10.0	12.0	22	29	17

* : Excludes Nagaland (Rural) due to part-receipt of returns.

N. A.: Not available due to part-receipt of returns.

Note : Infant mortality rates for Smaller States and Union Territories are for the period 1 997-99.

With compliments from Jayanat Kumar Banthia, Registrar General, India, 2-A Mansingh Road, New Delhi-110 011, India.
E-mail : orgindia @vsnl.net/ ((91) (11) 2338 3761 Fax : (91) (11) 2338 3145
Census and Vital Statistics Website on the Internet : http://www.censusindia.net

Table 2. Ninety five percent confidence limits (lower and upper limits) for

India/States/ Union Territories	*Birth Rate*						*Death*	
	Total		*Rural*		*Urban*		*Total*	
	Lower Limit	*Upper Limit*	*Lower Limit*	*Upper Limit*	*Lower Limit*	*Upper Limit*	*Lower Limit*	*Upper Limit*
1	*2*	*3*	*4*	*5*	*6*	*7*	*8*	*9*
India*	**24.7**	**25.2**	**26.4**	**26.9**	**19.4**	**20.5**	**8.0**	**8.2**
Bigger States								
1. Andhra Pradesh	20.1	21.3	20.4	21.8	18.2	20.4	7.7	8.4
2. Assam	25.6	27.6	26.4	28.7	17.2	19.4	8.6	9.8
3. Bihar	30.2	31.5	31.2	32.5	21.0	25.9	7.6	8.2
4. Gujarat	23.9	25.5	25.6	27.5	19.2	22.0	7.3	8.1
5. Haryana	25.3	27.8	26.0	29.2	21.1	24.1	6.7	7.4
6. Karnataka	21.3	22.8	22.5	24.4	17.7	20.0	6.9	7.6
7. Kerala	16.2	17.5	!6.3	17.7	15.0	17.7	6:0	6.7
8. Madhya Pradesh	29.6	31.2	31.3	33.2	21.4	24.0	9.4	10.3
9. Maharashtra	19.7	20.9	19.9	21.3	18.8	20.7	6.9	7.6
10. Orissa	22.4	24.0	22.8	24.5	18.4	20.8	9.4	10.2
11. Punjab	20.1	21.5	20.8	22.6	16.7	19.4	6.6	7.6

1	2	3	4	5	6	7	8	9
12. Rajasthan	29.7	31.4	30.9	32.9	23.0	25.4	7.4	8.1
13. Tamil Nadu	18.0	19.1	18.4	19.8	16.5	18.4	7.3	8.1
14. Uttar Pradesh	31.0	32.3	31.8	33.4	25.7	27.8	9.4	10.0
15. West Bengal	19.8	21.1	21.8	23.4	13.2	15.0	6.5	7.0
Smaller States								
1. Arunachal Pradesh	18.0	22.3	18.5	23.3	10.0	14.6		
2. Chhatisgarh	23.1	26.9	24.9	28.1	18.2	27.0		
3. Goa	13.1	14.9	13.1	15.6	12.0	14.9		
4. Jharkhand	23.7	29.0	27.1	30.0	10.2	27.7		
5. Himachal Pradesh	19.5	21.9	19.8	22.3	15.2	17.7		
6. Jammu & Kashmir	18.0	20.4	18.6	21.3	13.9	18.0		
7. Manipur	15.6	18.0	15.8	19.0	14.4	16.3		
8. Meghalaya	23.7	27.9	25.4	30.1	10.1	19.0		
9. Mizoram	15.4	18.3	19.7	22.0	9.6	14.5		
10. Nagaland	N.A.	N.A.	N.A.	N.A.	9.2	14.7		
11. Sikkim	20.7	23.1	21.0	23.5	11.0	15.9		
12. Tripura	12.6	17.2	12.6	18.0	10.5	16.1		
13. Uttaranchal	14.4	19.7	14.4	21.7	12.3	20.2		

1	2	3	4	5	6	7	8	9
Union Territories								
1. Andaman & Nicobar Islands	15.3	18.4	15.8	19.4	11.7	17.4		
2. Chandigarh	12.4	16.9	14.9	28.1	11.3	16.2		
3. Dadra & Nagar Haveli	12.1	48.7	11.1	51.6	17.4	23.3		
4. Daman & Diu	19.1	25.8	21.7	25.4	14.6	28.3		
5. Delhi	16.1	18.4	1 6.7	19.6	15.8	18.5		
6. Lakshadweep	15.8	22.7	16.3	24.1	15.3	21.4		
7. Pondicherry	16.4	19.4	16.3	19.9	15.4	19.9		

* Excludes Nagaland (Rural) due to part-receipt of returns.

N.A : Not available due to part-receipt of returns.

Note : Ninety five percent confidence limits for birth rate, death rate and infant mortality rate have been estimated using the formulae BR±2 S.E. (BR). DR±2 S.E. (DR) and IMR±2 S.E. (IMR) respectively.

Birth Rate, Death Rate and Infant Mortality Rate, 2002

Rate				*Infant Mortality Rate*						*India/States/ Union Territories*
Rural		*Urban*		*Total*		*Rural*		*Urban*		
Lower Limit	*Upper Limit*	*Lower Limit*	*Upper limit*	*Lower limit*	*Upper Limit*	*Lower limit*	*Upper limit*	*Lower limit*	*Upper limit*	
10	*11*	*12*	*13*	*14*	*15*	*16*	*17*	*18*	*19*	*1*
8.6	**8.9**	**5.9**	**6.3**	**62**	**65**	**68**	**71**	**36**	**43**	**India***
										Bigger States
8.5	9.3	5.0	6.1	57	68	64	77	25	45	1. Andhra Pradesh
8.9	10.2	5.1	6.9	64	77	66	80	27	50	2. Assam
7.8	8.5	5.5	6.7	56	65	57	66	38	62	3. Bihar
7.8	8.7	5.5	7.2	53	66	60	75	25	49	4. Gujarat
6.8	7.7	5.7	7.0	56	68	58	71	38	64	5. Haryana
7.5	8.3	5.1	6.4	50	59	59	71	17	33	6. Karnataka
6.0	6.8	5.4	7.1	7	13	7	14	2	13	7. Kerala
10.0	11.0	6.2	8.2	79	90	83	96	43	68	8. Madhya Pradesh
7.8	8.7	5.0	6.2	41	50	46	57	26	43	9. Maharashtra
9.8	10.7	5.7	7.1	79	95	82	99	45	67	10. Orissa
6.8	7.9	5.4	7.1	43	59	45	65	24	45	11. Punjab

10	11	12	13	14	15	16	17	18	19	1
7.6	8.4	5.5	7.2	73	83	76	87	41	69	12. Rajasthan
8.1	9.0	5.4	6.4	39	50	44	56	23	40	13. Tamil Nadu
9.9	10.6	6.7	7.9	76	83	80	87	50	65	14. Uttar Pradesh
6.6	7.2	5.9	6.9	44	54	46	57	28	44	15. West Bengal
										Smaller States
										1. Arunachal Pradesh
										2. Chhatisgarh
										3. Goa
										4. Jharkhand
										5. Himachal Pradesh
										6. Jammu & Kashmir
										7. Manipur
										8. Meghalaya
										9. Mizoram
										10. Nagaland
										11. Sikkim
										12. Tripura
										13. Uttaranchal

Confidence limits of Death Rate and Infant Mortality Rate for smaller States and Union territories have not been presented due to the small sample size and very large variations between the Upper and Lower tolerance limits.

1	*10*	*11*	*12*	*13*	*14*	*15*	*16*	*17*	*18*	*19*
Union territories										
1. Andaman & Nicobar Islands										
2. Chandigarh										
3. Dadra & Nagar Haveli										
4. Daman & Diu										
5. Delhi										
6. Lakshadweep										
7. Pondicherry										

Table 3: Death rate by sex and residence, 2002

India/States/ Union Territories	Total			Rural			Urban		
	Total	*Male*	*Female*	*Total*	*Male*	*Female*	*Total*	*Male*	*Female*
1	*2*	*3*	*4*	*5*	*6*	*7*	*8*	*9*	*10*
India*	**8.1**	**8.4**	**7.7**	**8.7**	**9.0**	**8.4**	**6.1**	**6.5**	**5.6**
Bigger States									
1. Andhra Pradesh	8.1	9.0	7.1	8.9	9.9	7.9	5.5	6.1	5.0
2. Assam	9.2	10.0	8.4	9.6	10.3	8.8	6.0	7.0	4.9
3. Bihar	7.9	7.6	8.3	8.2	7.7	8.6	6.1	6.5	5.6
4. Gujarat	7.7	8.3	7.0	8.3	8.9	7.6	6.4	7.2	5.5
5. Haryana	7.1	7.3	6.8	7.2	7.3	7.1	6.4	7.3	5.3
6. Karnataka	7.2	8.1	6.4	7.9	8.6	7.1	5.7	6.9	4.6
7. Kerala	6.4	7.5	5.3	6.4	7.5	5.4	6.2	7.6	5.0
8. Madhya Pradesh	9.8	9.9	9.7	10.5	10.6	10.3	7.2	7.1	7.4
9. Maharashtra	7.3	7.7	6.8	8.3	8.6	7.9	5.6	6.1	5.1
10. Orissa	9.8	10.3	9.4	10.3	10.7	9.8	6.4	7.0	5.8
11. Punjab	7.1	7.7	6.4	7.4	7.9	6.8	6.2	7.0	5.3
12. Rajasthan	7.7	7.9	7.4	8.0	8.2	7.7	6.4	6.7	6.0

1		2	3	4	5	6	7	8	9	10
13.	Tamil Nadu	7.7	8.3	7.1	8.6	9.4	7.7	5.9	6.2	5.7
14.	Uttar Pradesh	9.7	9.6	9.9	10.2	10.1	10.4	7.3	7.2	7.3
15.	West Bengal	6.7	7.0	6.5	6.9	7.1	6.7	6.4	6.8	5.9
Smaller States										
1.	Arunachal Pradesh	4.8	4.8	4.7	5.0	5.0	4.9	2.6	2.5	2.8
2.	Chhatisgarh	8.7	9.5	7.9	9.7	10.1	9.3	7.2	8.6	5.7
3.	Goa	8.3	9.7	6.9	9.0	11.2	6.9	7.2	7.6	6.8
4.	Jharkhand	7.9	8.5	7.4	8.6	9.2	7.9	5.8	6.2	5.4
5.	Himachal Pradesh	7.5	9.1	6.1	7.7	9.3	6.2	5.1	5.9	4.1
6.	Jammu & Kashmir	5.7	6.2	5.3	5.7	6.2	5.3	5.7	6.1	5.3
7.	Manipur	4.6	5.1	4.1	4.2	4.5	3.9	5.8	7.0	4.7
8.	Meghalaya	7.7	9.1	6.3	8.4	9.8	6.9	3.9	5.2	2.6
9.	Mizoram	4.8	6.2	3.5	5.7	7.4	4.0	3.7	4.7	2.8
10.	Nagaland	N.A.	N.A.	N.A.	N.A.	N.A.	N.A.	2.5	3.5	1.3
11.	Sikkim	4.9	4.9	4.9	5.0	5.0	4.9	4.1	3.7	4.5
12.	Tripura	5.7	6.4	5.1	5.6	6.3	5.0	6.2	6.9	5.6
13.	Uttaranchal	6.4	6.7	6.1	9.0	10.0	8.1	4.4	4.3	4.6

1	2	3	4	5	6	7	8	9	10
Union Territories									
1. Andaman & Nicobar Islands	5.5	5.9	5.2	6.1	6.2	6.0	3.8	4.9	2.6
2. Chandigarh	3.4	3.5	3.4	4.1	4.1	4.1	3.4	3.4	3.3
3. Dadra & Nagar Haveli	6.8	7.1	6.6	7.1	7.3	6.8	4.0	4.4	3.5
4. Daman & Diu	6.6	9.7	3.4	7.4	8.9	5.8	5.9	10.6	1.4
5. Delhi	5.1	5.2	5.1	5.7	5.6	5.9	5.1	5.1	4.9
6. Lakshadweep	5.2	4.8	5.7	5.3	4.2	6.4	5.1	5.3	4.9
7. Pondicherry	6.7	7.3	6.1	8.1	9.8	6.4	5.7	5.5	5.9

* Excludes Nagaland (Rural) due to part-receipt of returns.
N.A : Not available due to part-receipt of returns.
Note : Estimates of Death rate by sex are subject to year by year fluctuation.

Table 4 : Infant mortality rate by sex and residence, 2002

India/States/ Union Territories	*Total*			*Rural*			*Urban*		
	Total	*Male*	*Female*	*Total*	*Male*	*Female*	*Total*	*Male*	*Female*
1	*2*	*3*	*4*	*5*	*6*	*7*	*8*	*9*	*10*
India*	**63**	**62**	**65**	**69**	**67**	**72**	**40**	**40**	**39**
Bigger States									
1. Andhra Pradesh	62	64	60	71	69	72	35	47	23
2. Assam	70	70	71	73	72	73	38	34	43
3. Bihar	61	56	66	62	57	67	50	47	53
4. Gujarat	60	55	66	68	60	76	37	39	34
5. Haryana	62	54	73	64	56	75	51	43	61
6. Karnataka	55	56	53	65.	67	62	25	23	27
7. Kerala	10	9	12	11	8	14	8	11	4
8. Madhya Pradesh	85	81	88	89	85	94	56	60	51
9. Maharashtra	45	48	42	52	54	49	34	38	29
10. Orissa	87	95	79	90	101	80	56	45	69
11. Punjab	51	38	66	55	41	73	35	28	43
12. Rajasthan	78	75	80	81	79	83	55	49	62
13. Tamil Nadu	44	46	43	50	51	49	32	35	28

1	*2*	*3*	*4*	*5*	*6*	*7*	*8*	*9*	*10*
14. Uttar Pradesh	80	76	84	83	78	90	58	66	47
15. West Bengal	49	53	45	52	55	49	36	45	25
Smaller States									
1. Arunachal Pradesh	38	36	40	39	39	40	12	#	28
2. Chhatisgarh	64	61	66	73	84	62	46	17	72
3. Goa	16	17	16	18	18	19	13	15	10
4. Jharkhand	41	44	37	44	45	42	26	38	11
5. Himachal Pradesh	61	66	55	63	68	57	28	26	31
6. Jammu & Kashmir	43	45	40	45	46	44	28	38	18
7. Manipur	10	13	7	8	10	6	14	21	7
8. Meghalaya	66	64	69	68	60	75	51	105	#
9. Mizoram	5	9	2	1	#	3	14	27	#
10. Nagaland	N.A.	N.A.	N.A.	N.A.	N.A.	N.A.	20	#	43
11. Sikkim	25	23	27	25	23	27	13	n	26
12. Tripura	33	35	31	32	33	32	38	49	28
13. Uttaranchal	34	16	55	57	38	77	15	#	35
Union Territories									
1. Andaman & Nicobar Islands	23	17	29	27	17	38	7	14	#

	1	2	3	4	5	6	7	8	9	10
2.	Chandigarh	22	15	30	25	25	25	22	13	31
3.	Dadra & Nagar Haveli	51	51	52	53	53	52	26	#	54
4.	Daman & Diu	30	46	12	26	30	22	34	59	#
5.	Delhi	33	29	38	28	6	53	34	32	36
6.	Lakshadweep	15	6	26	18	11	25	12	#	26
7.	Pondicherry	25	24	25	32	34	29	20	17	22

* Excludes Nagaland (Rural) due to part-receipt of returns.

N.A. : Not available due to part receipt of returns.

\# : Inadequate sample to provide estimates.

Note : Estimates of Infant mortality rate by sex are subject to year by year fluctuations.

ABOUT THE SAMPLE REGISTRATION SYSTEM (SRS)

The Sample Registration System (SRS) is a large scale demographic survey for providing reliable annual estimates of birth rate, death rate and other fertility and mortality indicators at the national and sub-national levels. The vital rates in respect of the three newly created States of Chhatisgarh, Jharkhand and Uttaranchal are being presented since April, 2002 issue of SRS bulletin. The field investigation consists of continuous enumeration of births and deaths by a resident part time enumerator, generally a teacher and an independent survey every six months by a computer supervisor. The data obtained through these operations are matched. The unmatched and partially matched events are re-verified in the field and thereafter an unduplicated count of births and deaths is obtained. The SRS was initiated by the OFFICE OF THE REGISTRAR GENERAL, INDIA on a pilot basis in a few selected states in 1964-65 and it became fully operational during 1969-70 with about 3700 sample units. Thereafter the number of sample units was periodically increased. The sample unit in rural areas is a village or a segment of it if the village had a population of 1500 or more. In urban areas the sampling unit is a census enumeration block with a population ranging from 750 to 1000. At present SRS has 6671 sample units (4436 rural and 2235 urban) in all States and Union Territories covering about 1.1 million households and 6.41 million population.

Number of sample units and population covered India, States and Union Territories 2002

India/States/ Union Territories	*Number of sample units*			*Population covered (in '000)*		
	Total	*Rural*	*Urban*	*Total*	*Rural*	*Urban*
1	*2*	*3*	*4*	*5*	*6*	*7*
India	**6671**	**4436**	**2235**	**6407**	**5022**	**1385**
Bigger States						
1. Andhra Pradesh	310	210	100	311	243	67
2. Assam	275	200	75	250	206	44

1	2	3	4	5	6	7
3. Bihar	361	308	53	451	416	35
4. Gujarat	300	200	100	278	225	53
5. Haryana	180	110	70	216	165	52
6. Karnataka	375	260	115	365	290	75
7. Kerala	250	150	100	316	251	65
8. Madhya Pradesh	299	216	83	301	254	48
9. Maharashtra	375	200	175	345	241	104
10. Orissa	405	300	105	313	250	63
11. Punjab	200	120	80	177	129	48
12. Rajasthan	350	250	100	341	292	49
13. Tamil Nadu	375	200	175	355	237	118
14. Uttar Pradesh	615	428	187	663	561	102
15. West Bengal	475	300	175	481	372	109
Smaller States						
1. Arunachal Pradesh	56	50	6	47	40	7
2. Chhatisgarh	101	84	17	94	84	10
3. Goa	70	40	30	63	46	17
4. Jharkhand	139	92	47	122	97	24

1	2	3	4	5	6	7
5. Himachal Pradesh	190	140	50	103	74	28
6. Jammu & Kashmir	166	100	66	140	100	40
7. Manipur	150	100	50	138	101	37
8. Meghalaya	120	100	20	64	54	10
9. Mizoram	32	16	16	23	12	11
10. Nagaland	35	25	10	5	0	5
11. Sikkim	60	50	10	62	53	9
12. Tripura	75	60	15	89	80	9
13. Uttaranchal	35	22	13	31	25	6
Union Territories						
1. Andaman & Nicobar Islands	45	30	15	33	23	10
2. Chandigarh	30	5	25	28	8	20
3. Dadra & Nagar Haveli	25	20	5	28	24	4
4. Daman & Diu	17	15	2	21	19	1
5. Delhi	130	10	120	105	18	87
6. Lakshadweep	10	5	5	13	8	4
7. Pondicherry	40	20	20	36	23	13

Note : Total pollution may not add up to Rural and Urban population due to rounding.

SRS BULLETIN

SAMPLE REGISTRATION SYSTEM

REGISTRAR GENERAL, INDIA

Vital Statistics Division, West Block 1, Wing 1, 2nd Floor, R.K. Puram, New Delhi-110 066

Table 1. Estimate of Bith rate, Death rate, Natural growth rate and Infant mortality rate, 2003

India / States / Union Territories	*Birth rate*			*Death rate*			*Natural growth rate*			*Infant mortality rate*		
	Total	*Rural*	*Urban*	*Total*	*Rural*	*Urban*	*Total*	*Rural*	*Urban*	*Total*	*Rural*	*Urban*
1	*2*	*3*	*4*	*5*	*6*	*7*	*8*	*9*	*10*	*11*	*12*	*13*
India*	24.8	26.4	19.8	8.0	8.7	6.0	16.8	17.8	13.8	60	66	38
Bigger States												
1. Andhra Pradesh	20.4	20.9	19.1	8.0	8.8	5.4	12.5	12.1	13.7	59	67	33
2. Assam	26.3	27.2	18.0	9.1	9.5	5.9	17.2	17.7	12.0	67	70	35
3. Bihar	30.7	31.6	23.4	7.9	8.1	6.0	22.8	23.5	17.4	60	62	49
4. Gujarat	24.6	26.5	20.5	7.6	8.2	6.3	17.0	18.3	14.2	57	65	36
5. Haryana	26.3	27.4	22.3	7.1	7.3	6.2	19.3	20.1	16.1	59	61	49
6 Karnataka	21.8	23.2	18.6	7.2	7.8	5.6	14.6	15.3	13.0	52	61	24
7. Kerala	16.7	16.9	16.0	6.3	6.4	6.1	10.3	10.5	9.9	11	12	10
8. Madhya Pradesh	30.2	32.1	22.5	9.8	10.4	7.1	20.5	21.7	15.3	82	86	55

1		2	3	4	5	6	7	8	9	10	11	12	13
9.	Maharashtra	19.9	20.1	19.4	7.2	8.2	5.6	12.6	11.9	13.9	42	48	32
10.	Orissa	23.0	23.5	19.4	9.7	10.2	6.3	13.3	13.3	13.2	83	86	55
11.	Punjab	20.6	21.5	17.9	7.0	7.3	6.0	13.6	14.2	11.9	49	53	34
12.	Rajasthan	30.3	31.6	24.0	7.6	7.9	6.2	22.7	23.7	17.8	75	78	53
13.	Tamil Nadu	18.3	18.8	17.3	7.6	8.5	5.6	10.7	10.2	11.7	43	48	31
14.	Uttar Pradesh	31.3	32.2	26.6	9.5	10.1	7.0	21.7	22.2	19.7	76	79	55
15.	West Bengal	20.3	22.4	14.0	6.6	6.8	6.2	13.6	15.6	7.8	46	48	34
Smaller States													
1.	Arunachal Pradesh	18.9	19.5	12.3	4.7	4.9	2.5	14.2	14.6	9.8	34	35	11
2.	Chhatisgarh	25.2	26.8	22.5	8.5	9.5	7.1	16.6	17.3	15.5	70	77	55
3.	Goa	13.9	14.3	13.3	8.1	8.9	7.0	5.8	5.4	6.3	16	18	14
4.	Jharkhand	26.3	28.5	18.9	8.0	8.7	5.5	18.3	19.8	13.5	51	54	34
5.	Himachal Pradesh	20.6	20.9	16.1	7.1	7.3	4.9	13.5	13.6	11.2	49	51	26
6.	Jammu & Kashmir	18.6	19.2	15.9	5.7	5.9	5.3	12.9	13.4	10.6	44	46	32
7.	Manipur	15.5	16.1	14.1	4.8	4.9	4.4	10.7	11.1	9.7	16	15	19
8.	Meghalaya	24.7	26.6	13.8	7.4	8.1	3.4	17.3	18.5	10.4	57	59	44
9.	Mizoram	16.0	19.4	11.7	5.1	6.2	3.6	10.9	13.2	8.1	16	18	14
10.	Nagaland	N.A.	N.A.	11.8	N.A.	N.A.	2.4	N.A.	N.A.	9.5	N.A.	N.A.	16

1		2	3	4	5	6	7	8	9	10	11	12	13
11.	Sikkim	21.9	22.3	13.4	5.0	5.1	4.0	16.9	17.2	9.5	33	33	23
12.	Tripura	14.5	14.8	13.2	5.5	5.4	6.0	9.0	9.4	7.2	32	32	31
13.	Uttaranchal	17.2	18.9	16.0	6.5	8.6	4.8	10.8	10.3	11.1	41	62	21
Union Territories													
1.	Andaman & Nicobar Islands	17.1	18.1	14.3	5.6	6.4	3.4	11.6	11.8	11.0	18	20	11
2.	Chandigarh	14.8	22.4	13.9	3.8	3.9	3.8	11.0	18.4	10.1	19	25	18
3.	Dadra & Nagar Haveli	30.3	31.2	20.1	6.1	6.4	3.4	24.1	24.8	16.7	54	57	19
4.	Daman & Diu	22.4	23.3	21.6	6.6	7.3	6.0	15.8	16.0	15.6	39	41	38
5.	Delhi	17.3	21.3	16.8	5.0	5.5	4.9	12.4	15.8	11.9	28	32	28
6.	Lakshadweep	19.0	20.1	18.0	5.2	5.0	5.4	13.8	15.1	12.6	26	31	21
7.	Pondicherry	17.5	18.0	17.1	6.3	7.7	5.4	11.2	10.3	11.8	24	33	17

* Excludes Nagaland (Rural) due to part-receipt of returns.
N.A.: Not available due to part-receipt of returns.
Note : Infant mortality rates for Smaller States and Union Territories are based on three-years 2001-03.

Published and issued by office of the, Registrar General, India, 2-A Mansingh Road, New Delhi-110 011, India.
E-mail : orgindia @vsnl.net Phone : ((91) (11) 2338 3761 Fax : (91) (11) 2338 3145.
Census and Vital Statistics Website on the Internet : http://www.censusindia.net.

Table 2. Ninety five percent confidence limits (lower and upper limits) for

India/States/ Union Territories	Birth Rate						Death	
	Total		Rural		Urban		Total	
	Lower Limit	Upper Limit	Lower Limit	Upper limit	Lower limit	Upper Limit	Lower limit	Upper limit
1	2	3	4	5	6	7	8	9
India*	**24.5**	**25.1**	**26.0**	**26.8**	**19.2**	**20.4**	**7.9**	**8.1**
Bigger States								
1. Andhra Pradesh	19.7	21.2	20.0	21.7	17.8	20.5	7.6	8.3
2. Assam	25.5	27.1	26.4	28.1	16.5	19.4	8.6	9.6
3. Bihar	30.0	31.3	31.1	32.1	20.0	26.8	7.6	8.2
4. Gujarat	23.7	25.5	25.5	27.6	19.0	22.1	7.2	8.0
5. Haryana	25.3	27.3	26.2	28.5	20.3	24.3	6.6	7.6
6. Karnataka	21.0	22.5	22.4	24.0	16.9	20.2	6.8	7.5
7. Kerala	16.1	17.3	16.2	17.6	14.8	17.2	6.0	6.6
8. Madhya Pradesh	29.5	30.9	31.4	32.9	20.7	24.2	9.5	10.1
9. Maharashtra	19.3	20.5	19.5	20.8	18.3	20.6	6.9	7.5
10. Orissa	22.3	23.7	22.7	24.2	18.1	20.7	9.3	10.1
11. Punjab	19.9	21.3	20.8	22.2	16.3	19.5	6.6	7.4

1		*2*	*3*	*4*	*5*	*6*	*7*	*8*	*9*
12.	Rajasthan	29.5	31.1	30.7	32.4	22.5	25.6	7.3	7.9
13.	Tamil Nadu	17.8	18.8	18.2	19.4	16.2	18.4	7.3	7.9
14.	Uttar Pradesh	29.8	32.8	30.5	34.0	24.9	28.3	9.0	10.0
15.	West Bengal	19.7	20.8	21.7	23.1	12.9	15.0	6.4	6.8
Smaller States									
1.	Arunachal Pradesh	16.3	21.5	16.6	22.4	6.6	18.0		
2.	Chhatisgarh	23.4	26.9	25.4	28.3	18.2	26.9		
3.	Goa	13.0	14.7	13.3	15.2	11.7	14.9		
4.	Jharkhand	23.4	29.2	26.9	30.1	9.2	28.7		
5.	Himachal Pradesh	19.4	21.8	19.7	22.2	14.1	18.2		
6.	Jammu & Kashmir	17.4	19.8	17.9	20.6	14.1	17.6		
7.	Manipur	14.6	16.5	14.9	17.2	12.0	16.2		
8.	Meghalaya	22.9	26.5	24.6	28.5	11.3	16.3		
9.	Mizoram	14.0	18.0	16.8	22.1	8.7	14.7		
10.	Nagaland	N.A.	N.A.	N.A.	N.A.	10.7	12.9		
11.	Sikkim	20.9	23.0	21.1	23.4	10.3	16.6		
12.	Tripura	13.0	16.0	13.0	16.5	11.5	14.8		
13.	Uttaranchal	15.2	19.3	16.0	21.8	13.0	19.0		

1	2	3	4	5	6	7	8	9
Union Territories								
1. Andaman & Nicobar Islands	15.6	18.6	16.2	20.0	12.4	16.3		
2. Chandigarh	12.6	17.1	17.8	26.9	11.4	16.4		
3. Dadra & Nagar Haveli	27.6	33.0	28.3	34.1	17.7	22.5		
4. Daman & Diu	11.2	33.6	21.4	25.2	2.5	40.6		
5. Delhi	16.2	18.5	18.8	23.9	15.5	18.1		
6. Lakshadweep	17.0	21.1	17.7	22.6	14.6	21.3		
7. Pondicherry	15.7	19.3	16.5	19.6	14.2	20.0		

* Excludes Nagaland (Rural) due to part-receipt of returns.

N.A : Not available due to part-receipt of returns.

Note : Ninety five percent confidence limits for birth rate, death rate and infant mortality rate have been estimated using the formulae BR±2 S.E. (BR), DR±2 S.E. (DR) and IMR+2 S.E. (IMR) respectively.

Birth Rate, Death Rate and Infant Mortality Rate, 2002

Rate				*Infant Mortality Rate*						
Rural		*Urban*		*Total*		*Rural*		*Urban*		*India/States/ Union Territories*
Lower Limit	*Upper Limit*	*Lower Limit*	*Upper Limit*	*Lower Limit*	*Upper Limit*	*Lower Limit*	*Upper Limit*	*Lower Limit*	*Upper Limit*	
10	*11*	*12*	*13*	*14*	*15*	*16*	*17*	*18*	*19*	*1*
8.5	**8.8**	**5.8**	**6.2**	**59**	**62**	**64**	**68**	**35**	**41**	**India***
										Bigger States
8.4	9.2	4.7	6.1	54	64	61	72	26	39	1. Andhra Pradesh
8.9	10.0	5.2	6.7	59	75	61	78	25	45	2. Assam
7.8	8.4	4.9	7.1	56	64	57	66	38	59	3. Bihar
7.7	8.7	5.7	6.9	52	62	59	70	27	44	4. Gujarat
6.7	7.9	5.5	6.8	51	66	52	70	40	57	5. Haryana
7.5	8.2	5.0	6.2	46	57	54	69	18	30	6. Karnataka
6.0	6.7	5.5	6.7	9	14	9	15	4	16	7. Kerala
10.1	10.8	6.4	7.9	76	88	79	93	45	65	8. Madhya Pradesh
7.8	8.5	5.1	6.1	38	46	43	52	25	39	9. Maharashtra
9.7	10.6	5.6	6.9	76	89	78	93	43	66	10. Orissa
6.9	7.8	5.3	6.7	42	56	44	61	25	44	11. Punjab

10	11	12	13	14	15	16	17	18	19	1
7.5	8.2	5.5	6.9	71	79	74	82	42	64	12. Rajasthan
8.2	8.9	5.1	6.1	39	47	43	53	24	38	13. Tamil Nadu
9.5	10.7	6.4	7.6	71	80	74	84	49	62	14. Uttar Pradesh
6.5	7.0	5.7	6.7	42	50	44	53	26	41	15. West Bengal
										Smaller States
										1. Arunachal Pradesh
										2. Chhatisgarh
										3. Goa
										4. Jharkhand
										5. Himachal Pradesh
										6. Jammu & Kashmir
										7. Manipur
										8. Meghalaya
										9. Mizoram
										10. Nagaland
										11. Sikkim
										12. Tripura
										13. Uttaranchal

Confidence limits of Death Rate and Infant Mortality Rate for smaller States and Union Territories have not been presented due to the small sample size and very large variations between the Upper and Lower tolerance limits.

10	11	12	13	14	15	16	17	18	19	1
										Union Territories
										1. Andaman & Nicobar Islands
										2. Chandigarh
										3. Dadra & Nagar Haveli
										4. Daman & Diu
										5. Delhi
										6. Lakshadweep
										7. Pondicherry

Table 3. Death rate by sex and residence, 2003

India/States/ Union Territories	*Total*			*Rural*			*Urban*		
	Total	*Male*	*Female*	*Total*	*Male*	*Female*	*Total*	*Male*	*Female*
1	*2*	*3*	*4*	*5*	*6*	*7*	*8*	*9*	*10*
India*	**8.0**	**8.4**	**7.5**	**8.7**	**9.1**	**8.2**	**6.0**	**6.4**	**5.4**
Bigger States									
1. Andhra Pradesh	8.0	8.9	7.0	8.8	9.9	7.8	5.4	6.0	4.8
2. Assam	9.1	9.2	9.1	9.5	9.5	9.5	5.9	6.5	5.3
3. Bihar	7.9	7.6	8.2	8.1	7.8	8.4	6.0	5.8	6.2
4. Gujarat	7.6	8.3	6.9	8.2	9.0	7.4	6.3	6.8	5.8
5. Haryana	7.1	8.0	6.0	7.3	8.4	6.1	6.2	6.7	5.5
6. Karnataka	7.2	7.9	6.5	7.8	8.7	7.0	5.6	6.0	5.2
7. Kerala	6.3	7.2	5.5	6.4	7.3	5.5	6.1	6.8	5.5
8. Madhya Pradesh	9.8	10.2	9.3	10.4	10.8	9.9	7.1	7.5	6.8
9. Maharashtra	7.2	7.7	6.7	8.2	8.7	7.6	5.6	6.1	5.0
10. Orissa	9.7	10.3	9.1	10.2	10.8	9.6	6.3	7.1	5.3
11. Punjab	7.0	7.6	6.4	7.3	8.0	6.7	6.0	6.5	5.4
12. Rajasthan	7.6	8.2	6.9	7.9	8.5	7.2	6.2	6.8	5.6
13. Tamil Nadu	7.6	8.1	7.0	8.5	9.0	8.1	5.6	6.4	4.8

1	*2*	*3*	*4*	*5*	*6*	*7*	*8*	*9*	*10*
14. Uttar Pradesh	9.5	9.7	9.4	10.1	10.2	9.9	7.0	7.0	6.9
15. West Bengal	6.6	7.2	6.0	6.8	7.4	6.1	6.2	6.7	5.6
Smaller States									
1. Arunachal Pradesh	4.7	4.5	4.9	4.9	4.7	5.1	2.5	2.2	2.7
2. Chhatisgarh	8.5	9.1	8.0	9.5	10.1	8.9	7.1	7.6	6.5
3. Goa	8.1	8.9	7.3	8.9	10.0	7.8	7.0	7.4	6.5
4. Jharkhand	8.0	7.7	8.2	8.7	8.4	9.0	5.5	5.6	5.3
5. Himachal Pradesh	7.1	8.3	6.0	7.3	8.6	6.1	4.9	5.6	4.2
6. Jammu & Kashmir	5.7	6.6	4.8	5.9	6.7	5.0	5.3	6.1	4.3
7. Manipur	4.8	5.6	4.0	4.9	5.9	4.0	4.4	4.7	4.0
8. Meghalaya	7.4	7.5	7.2	8.1	7.9	8.2	3.4	5.0	1.8
9. Mizoram	5.1	6.8	3.4	6.2	8.4	4.1	3.6	4.8	2.5
10. Nagaland	N.A.	N.A.	N.A.	N.A.	N.A.	N.A.	2.4	3.3	1.3
11. Sikkim	5.0	5.5	4.6	5.1	5.5	4.6	4.0	5.5	2.2
12. Tripura	5.5	6.5	4.5	5.4	6.3	4.4	6.0	7.3	4.8
13. Uttaranchal	6.5	7.4	5.5	8.6	9.4	7.9	4.8	5.8	3.7

1	2	3	4	5	6	7	8	9	10
Union Territories									
1. Andaman & Nicobar Islands	5.6	7.3	3.7	6.4	7.9	4.7	3.4	4.3	2.3
2. Chandigarh	3.8	3.8	3.9	3.9	4.2	3.6	3.8	3.7	3.9
3. Dadra & Nagar Haveli	6.1	7.7	4.6	6.4	8.1	4.7	3.4	3.4	3.4
4. Daman & Diu	6.6	6.6	6.6	7.3	8.7	5.8	6.0	4.6	7.3
5. Delhi	5.0	5.5	4.4	5.5	6.2	4.8	4.9	5.4	4.3
6. Lakshadweep	5.2	5.5	4.9	5.0	5.1	4.9	5.4	5.8	5.0
7. Pondicherry	6.3	7.6	5.1	7.7	9.7	5.8	5.4	6.2	4.6

* Excludes Nagaland (Rural) due to part-receipt of returns.

N.A : Not available due to part-receipt of returns.

Note : Estimates of Death rate by sex are subject to year by year fluctuation.

Table 4. Infant mortality rate by sex and residence, 2003

India/States/ Union Territories	*Total*			*Rural*			*Urban*		
	Total	*Male*	*Female*	*Total*	*Male*	*Female*	*Total*	*Male*	*Female*
1	*2*	*3*	*4*	*5*	*6*	*7*	*8*	*9*	*10*
India*	60	57	64	66	63	69	38	33	44
Bigger States									
1. Andhra Pradesh	59	59	59	67	65	68	33	36	30
2. Assam	67	69	65	70	72	67	35	29	40
3. Bihar	60	59	62	62	59	65	49	59	37
4. Gujarat	57	54	61	65	63	67	36	28	44
5. Haryana	59	54	65	61	56	67	49	43	56
6. Karnataka	52	51	52	61	62	61	24	20	29
7. Kerala	11	11	12	12	12	12	10	8	12
8. Madhya Pradesh	82	77	86	86	85	87	55	32	79
9. Maharashtra	42	32	54	48	37	60	32	23	43
10. Orissa	83	82	83	86	86	85	55	50	61
11. Punjab	49	46	52	53	49	57	34	33	36
12. Rajasthan	75	70	81	78	72	86	53	58	47
13. Tamil Nadu	43	44	41	48	50	46	31	32	31

	1	2	3	4	5	6	7	8	9	10
14.	Uttar Pradesh	76	69	84	79	71	88	55	54	57
15.	West Bengal	46	45	46	48	48	48	34	32	35
Smaller States										
1.	Arunachal Pradesh	34	31	38						
2.	Chhattisgarh	70	68	71						
3.	Goa	16	15	18						
4.	Jharkhand	51	50	52						
5.	Himachal Pradesh	49	54	44						
6.	Jammu & Kashmir	44	46	41						
7.	Manipur	16	18	13						
8.	Meghalaya	57	56	59						
9.	Mizoram	16	16	17	Infant mortality rates for smaller States and Union Territories are based on three-years period 2001-03. On account of wide year-to-year fluctuations due to inadequate sample size, the infant mortality rate by sex separately for rural and urban areas is not given.					
10.	Nagaland	N.A.	N.A.	N.A.						
11.	Sikkim	33	34	31						
12.	Tripura	32	36	27						
13.	Uttaranchal	41	31	53						

1		2	3	4	5	6	7	8	9	10
Union Territories										
1.	Andaman & Nicobar Islands	18	12	24						
2.	Chandigarh	19	21	16						
3.	Dadra & Nagar Haveli	54	69	39						
4.	Daman & Diu	39	43	34						
5.	Delhi	28	28	29						
6.	Lakshadweep	26	21	32						
7.	Pondicherry	24	29	18						

* : Excludes Nagaland (Rural) due to part-receipt of returns.

N.A. : Not available due to part receipt of returns.

Note : Infant mortality rates for smaller States and Union Territories are based on three-years period 2001-03. Due to inadequate sample size, rural and urban breakup of infant mortality rate is not given.

ABOUT THE SAMPLE REGISTRATION SYSTEM (SRS)

The Sample Registration System (SRS) is a large-scale demographic survey for providing reliable annual estimates of birth rate, death rate and other fertility and mortality indicators at the national and sub-national levels. The vital rates in respect of the three newly created States of Chhatisgarh, Jharkhand and Uttaranchal are being presented since April 2002 issue of SRS bulletin. The field investigation consists of continuous enumeration of births and deaths by a resident part time enumerator, generally a teacher and an independent survey every six months by a computer supervisor. The data obtained through these operations are matched. The unmatched and partially matched events are re-verified in the field and thereafter an unduplicated count of births and deaths is obtained. The SRS was initiated by the OFFICE OF THE REGISTRAR GENERAL, INDIA on a pilot basis in a few selected states in 1964-65 and it became fully operational during 1969-70 with about 3700 sample units. Thereafter the number of sample units was periodically increased. The sample unit in rural areas is a village or a segment of it if the village had a population of 1500 or more. In urban areas the sampling unit is a census enumeration block with a population ranging from 750 to 1000. At present SRS has 6671 sample units (4436 rural and 2235 urban) in all States and Union territories. However, the vital rates provided in this Bulletin is based on 6645 sample units (4410 rural and 2235 urban covering about 1.1 million households and 6.45 million population. Data for 1 rural in Madhya Pradesh and 25 rural units in Nagaland could not be included due to various reasons.

Number of sample units and population covered India, States and Union Territories, 2003

India/States/ Union Territories	*Number of sample units*			*Population covered (in '000)*		
	Total	*Rural*	*Urban*	*Total*	*Rural*	*Urban*
1	*2*	*3*	*4*	*5*	*6*	*7*
India	**6645**	**4410**	**2235**	**6452**	**5064**	**1387**
Bigger States						
1. Andhra Pradesh	310	210	100	310	243	67

1	2	3	4	5	6	7
2. Assam	275	200	75	252	208	44
3. Bihar	361	308	53	457	422	35
4. Gujarat	300	200	100	280	227	53
5. Haryana	180	110	70	217	165	52
6. Karnataka	375	260	115	364	289	75
7. Kerala	250	150	100	319	254	65
8. Madhya Pradesh	299	215	82	302	254	48
9. Maharashtra	375	200	175	345	241	103
10. Orissa	405	300	105	314	251	63
11. Punjab	200	120	80	178	130	48
12. Rajasthan	350	250	100	345	296	49
13. Tamil Nadu	375	200	175	355	237	118
14. Uttar Pradesh	615	428	187	671	568	103
15. West Bengal	475	300	175	485	377	109
Smaller States						
1. Arunachal Pradesh	56	50	6	48	41	7
2. Chhattisgarh	101	84	18	95	84	10
3. Goa	70	40	30	63	45	17

1		2	3	4	5	6	7
4.	Jharkhand	139	92	47	124	99	25
5.	Himachal Pradesh	190	140	50	103	75	28
6.	Jammu & Kashmir	166	100	66	141	101	40
7.	Manipur	150	100	50	139	102	37
8.	Meghalaya	120	100	20	65	56	10
9.	Mizoram	32	16	16	23	12	11
10.	Nagaland	10	0	10	5	0	5
11.	Sikkim	60	50	10	63	54	9
12.	Tripura	75	60	15	89	80	9
13.	Uttaranchal	35	22	13	31	25	6
Union Territories							
1.	Andaman & Nicobar Islands	45	30	15	33	23	10
2.	Chandigarh	30	5	25	29	8	21
3.	Dadra & Nagar Haveli	25	20	5	29	25	4
4.	Daman & Diu	17	15	2	21	20	1
5.	Delhi	130	10	120	107	18	89
6.	Lakshadweep	10	5	5	13	9	4
7.	Pondicherry	40	20	20	36	23	13

Note: Total population may not add up to Rural and Urban population due to rounding.

SRS BULLETIN
SAMPLE REGISTRATION SYSTEM
REGISTRAR GENERAL, INDIA
Vital Statistics Division, West Block 1, Wing 1, 2nd Floor, R.K. Puram, New Delhi-110 066

Table 1. Estimates of Birth rate, Death Rate, Natural growth rate and Infant mortality rate, 2005

India / States / Union Territories	*Birth rate*			*Death rate*			*Natural growth rate*			*Infant mortality rate*		
	Total	*Rural*	*Urban*	*Total*	*Rural*	*Urban*	*Total*	*Rural*	*Urban*	*Total*	*Rural*	*Urban*
1	*2*	*3*	*4*	*5*	*6*	*7*	*8*	*9*	*10*	*11*	*12*	*13*
India	**23.8**	**25.6**	**19.1**	**7.6**	**8.1**	**6.0**	**16.3**	**17.5**	**13.1**	**58**	**64**	**40**
Bigger states												
1. Andhra Pradesh	19.1	20.1	16.7	7.3	7.9	5.9	11.8	12.2	10.8	57	63	39
2. Assam	25.0	26.6	15.3	8.7	9.2	5.6	16.3	17.4	9.6	68	71	39
3. Bihar	30.4	31.2	23.8	8.1	8.3	6.6	22.3	22.9	17.2	61	62	47
4. Chhattisgarh	27.2	29.0	20.0	8.1	8.4	6.9	19.1	20.6	13.1	63	65	52
5. Delhi	18.6	19.0	18.5	4.6	5.5	4.5	13.9	13.5	14.0	35	44	33
6. Gujarat	23.7	25.5	21.0	7.1	8.0	5.8	16.6	17.5	15.2	54	63	37
7. Haryana	24.3	25.7	21.0	6.7	7.0	5.8	17.6	18.7	15.1	60	64	45
8. Jammu & Kashmir	18.9	20.2	14.3	5.5	5.7	5.0	13.4	14.6	9.3	50	53	39

1	2	3	4	5	6	7	8	9	10	11	12	13
9. Jharkhand	26.8	28.8	18.7	7.9	8.4	5.7	18.9	20.4	13.0	50	53	33
10. Karnataka	20.6	22.1	17.9	7.1	7.9	5.6	13.5	14.2	12.3	50	54	39
11. Kerala	15.0	15.1	14.8	6.4	6.3	6.5	8.7	8.8	8.2	14	15	12
12. Madhya Pradesh	29.4	31.6	22.0	9.0	9.8	6.1	20.5	21.8	16.0	76	80	54
13. Maharashtra	19.0	19.6	18.2	6.7	7.4	5.7	12.3	12.2	12.5	36	41	27
14. Orissa	22.3	23.2	16.3	9.5	9.9	7.0	12.8	13.4	9.3	75	78	55
15. Punjab	18.1	18.8	17.0	6.7	7.2	5.8	11.4	11.6	11.2	44	49	37
16. Rajasthan	28.6	30.2	23.8	7.0	7.2	6.2	21.6	22.9	17.6	68	75	43
17. Tamil Nadu	16.5	16.9	16.0	7.4	8.2	6.2	9.2	8.7	9.8	37	39	34
18. Uttar Pradesh	30.4	31.3	26.5	8.7	9.1	6.8	21.7	22.2	19.7	73	77	54
19. West Bengal	18.8	21.2	12.6	6.4	6.3	6.6	12.4	14.9	6.0	38	40	31
Smaller States												
1. Arunachal Pradesh	23.3	24.4	18.7	5.0	5.5	2.8	18.3	18.9	15.9	37	39	17
2. Goa	14.8	13.9	15.4	7.1	8.9	5.8	7.7	5.0	9.5	16	16	15
3. Himachal Pradesh	20.0	20.7	13.3	6.9	7.1	4.7	13.1	13.6	8.6	49	50	20
4. Manipur	14.7	14.5	15.5	4.1	4.0	4.4	10.7	10.5	11.1	13	12	14
5. Meghalaya	25.1	27.3	15.1	7.5	7.9	6.0	17.5	19.4	9.1	49	50	42
6. Mizoram	18.8	23.2	14.4	5.1	6.2	4.1	13.7	17.1	10.3	20	26	10

1	2	3	4	5	6	7	8	9	10	11	12	13
7. Nagaland	16.4	16.5	16.1	3.8	4.0	3.1	12.6	12.5	13.1	18	17	22
8. Sikkim	19.9	20.2	18.0	5.1	5.2	4.8	14.8	15.0	13.2	30	31	15
9. Tripura	16.0	16.5	13.8	5.7	5.7	5.8	10.3	10.7	8.0	31	31	29
10. Uttaranchal	20.9	22.1	16.6	7.4	7.9	5.3	13.6	14.2	11.2	42	56	19
Union Territories												
1. Andaman & Nicobar Islands	15.7	17.5	12.6	4.7	5.3	3.6	11.1	12.2	9.0	27	30	18
2. Chandigarh	17.3	23.3	16.7	4.5	2.7	4.7	12.7	20.6	12.0	19	25	18
3. Dadra & Nagar Haveli	29.4	29.2	30.0	5.1	5.6	3.1	24.3	23.6	26.8	42	45	29
4. Daman & Diu	19.1	20.6	16.8	5.6	5.3	6.1	13.5	15.3	10.6	28	32	21
5. Lakshadweep	19.1	19.0	19.2	6.3	7.5	5.2	12.7	11.4	14.0	22	17	27
6. Pondicherry	16.2	16.9	15.8	7.1	8.0	6.7	9.0	9.0	9.1	28	38	22

Note: Infant mortality rates for smaller States and Union Territories are based on three-years period 2003-05.

Published and issued by Office of the Registrar General, India, 2-A Mansingh Road, New Delhi 110 011, India.
E mail: orgindia @ vsnl.net Phone: (91) (11) 2338 3761 Fax: (91) (11) 2338 3145
Census and Vital Statistics Website on the Internet: http://www.censusindia.net

Table 2. Ninety five percent confidence limits (lower and upper limits) for

India/States/ Union Territories	*Birth Rate*						*Death*	
	Total		*Rural*		*Urban*		*Total*	
	Lower Limit	*Upper Limit*	*Lower Limit*	*Upper Limit*	*Lower Limit*	*Upper Limit*	*Lower Limit*	*Upper Limit*
1	*2*	*3*	*4*	*5*	*6*	*7*	*8*	*9*
India	**23.6**	**24.1**	**25.3**	**25.9**	**18.8**	**19.4**	**7.4**	**7.7**
Bigger States								
1. Andhra Pradesh	18.3	19.9	19.1	21.1	15.5	17.8	6.9	7.8
2. Assam	23.0	26.9	24.4	28.8	14.3	16.3	8.0	9.3
3. Bihar	29.8	31.1	30.5	31.9	22.3	25.2	7.7	8.5
4. Chhattisgarh	24.8	29.6	25.9	32.0	18.4	21.7	7.2	9.0
5. Delhi	17.5	19.7	15.7	22.2	17.3	19.7	4.2	5.0
6. Gujarat	22.7	24.7	24.2	26.8	19.4	22.6	6.8	7.5
7. Haryana	22.9	25.6	24.0	27.4	19.1	22.8	6.2	7.1
8. Jammu & Kashmir	17.9	20.0	18.9	21.6	13.0	15.7	5.1	5.9
9. Jharkhand	25.4	28.2	27.1	30.5	17.5	19.9	7.3	8.4
10. Karnataka	19.6	21.6	20.7	23.5	16.6	19.2	6.6	7.5
11. Kerala	14.4	15.7	14.4	15.8	13.6	15.9	6.1	6.7

1	2	3	4	5	6	7	8	9
12. Madhya Pradesh	28.2	30.6	30.2	33.1	20.4	23.7	8.5	9.4
13. Maharashtra	18.5	19.5	19.1	20.2	17.2	19.2	6.4	6.9
14. Orissa	21.4	23.1	22.3	24.2	15.2	17.5	9.0	9.9
15. Punjab	17.4	18.8	17.9	19.7	15.9	18.1	6.3	7.1
16. Rajasthan	27.5	29.6	29.0	31.3	21.7	25.9	6.6	7.4
17. Tamil Nadu	16.0	17.0	16.2	17.5	15.3	16.7	7.0	7.7
18. Uttar Pradesh	29.5	31.2	30.3	32.3	25.2	27.8	8.3	9.0
19. West Bengal	18.1	19.5	20.3	22.1	11.8	13.4	6.1	6.7
Smaller States								
1. Arunachal Pradesh	19.9	26.7	20.3	28.6	13.8	23.6		
2. Goa	13.3	16.3	12.9	14.9	12.9	17.8		
3. Himachal Pradesh	18.7	21.2	19.3	22.1	11.8	14.8		
4. Manipur	13.7	15.8	13.3	15.6	13.1	17.9		
5. Meghalaya	22.7	27.4	24.5	30.1	11.9	18.3		
6. Mizoram	16.5	21.2	19.5	26.9	11.6	17.2		
7. Nagaland	14.5	18.3	14.2	18.7	12.4	19.9		
8. Sikkim	18.3	21.5	18.5	21.9	14.4	21.6		
9. Tripura	14.9	17.1	15.3	17.6	11.3	16.3		
10. Uttaranchal	16.8	25.0	16.7	27.4	14.6	18.6		

1	2	3	4	5	6	7	8	9
Union Territories								
1. Andaman & Nicobar Islands	14.0	17.5	15.6	19.4	9.2	16.0		
2. Chandigarh	14.7	19.8	19.7	26.9	14.0	19.5		
3. Dadra & Nagar Haveli	26.9	31.9	26.5	32.0	23.7	36.2		
4. Daman & Diu	16.6	21.5	17.8	23.3	12.3	21.2		
5. Lakshadweep	16.6	21.5	14.7	23.2	16.8	21.6		
6. Pondicherry	14.9	17.4	15.4	18.4	14.0	17.5		

Note : Ninety five percent confidence limits for Birth rate, Death rate and Infant mortality rate have been estimated using the formulae BR ± 2 S.E.(BR), DR ± 2 S.E.(DR) and IMR ± 2 S.E.(IMR) respectively.

Birth Rate, Death Rate and Infant Mortality Rate, 2005

Death Rate				*Infant Morrtality Rate*						
Rural		*Urban*		*Total*		*Rural*		*Urban*		*India/States/ Union Territories*
Lower Limit	*Upper Limit*	*Lower Limit*	*Upper Limit*	*Lower Limit*	*Upper Limit*	*Lower Limit*	*Upper Limit*	*Lower Limit*	*Upper Limit*	
10	*11*	*12*	*13*	*14*	*15*	*16*	*17*	*18*	*19*	*1*
8.0	**8.2**	**5.9**	**6.2**	**57**	**60**	**62**	**66**	**38**	**42**	**India**
										Bigger States
7.4	8.5	5.3	6.5	51	63	56	70	32	47	1. Andhra Pradesh
8.4	9.9	5.1	6.2	61	75	63	78	32	47	2. Assam
7.9	8.7	6.0	7.2	56	66	57	68	40	55	3. Bihar
7.3	9.4	6.1	7.8	55	72	56	75	45	59	4. Chhattisgarh
4.2	6.8	4.1	4.9	29	41	29	59	27	40	5. Delhi
7.6	8.5	5.1	6.5	48	59	55	70	28	46	6. Gujarat
6.5	7.6	5.1	6.5	54	65	57	72	39	52	7. Haryana
5.2	6.1	4.3	5.7	44	56	46	60	26	52	8. Jammu & Kashmir
7.7	9.1	5.0	6.4	44	57	45	61	23	43	9. Jharkhand
7.4	8.4	4.9	6.3	44	55	47	62	32	46	10. Karnataka
6.0	6.7	5.9	7.2	10	19	10	21	4	20	11. Kerala

10	11	12	13	14	15	16	17	18	19	1
9.3	10.4	5.4	6.7	69	82	72	88	45	62	12. Madhya Pradesh
7.2	7.7	5.3	6.1	32	39	37	46	20	34	13. Maharashtra
9.4	10.3	6.2	7.9	68	83	69	86	45	65	14. Orissa
6.7	7.7	5.2	6.5	38	51	40	57	29	45	15. Punjab
6.8	7.7	5.6	6.9	61	74	67	82	34	51	16. Rajasthan
7.8	8.6	5.7	6.7	33	41	34	44	27	41	17. Tamil Nadu
8.7	9.5	6.1	7.4	69	77	72	82	49	58	18. Uttar Pradesh
5.9	6.6	6.1	7.1	34	43	35	45	24	39	19. West Bengal
										Smaller States
										1. Arunachal Pradesh
										2. Goa
										3. Himachal Pradesh
										4. Manipur
										5. Meghalaya
										6. Mizoram
										7. Nagaland
										8. Sikkim
										9. Tripura
										10. Uttaranchal

Confidence limits of Death Rate and Infant Mortality Rate for smaller States and Union Territories have not been presented due to the small sample size and very large variations between the Upper and Lower tolerance limits.

1	10	11	12	13	14	15	16	17	18	19
Union Territories										
1. Andaman & Nicobar Islands										
2. Chandigarh										
3. Dadra & Nagar Haveli										
4. Daman & Diu										
5. Lakshadweep										
6. Pondicherry										

Table 3. Death rate by sex and residence, 2005

India/States/ Union Territories	*Total*			*Rural*			*Urban*		
	Total	*Male*	*Female*	*Total*	*Male*	*Female*	*Total*	*Male*	*Female*
1	*2*	*3*	*4*	*5*	*6*	*7*	*8*	*9*	*10*
India	**7.6**	**8.0**	**7.1**	**8.1**	**8.5**	**7.7**	**6.0**	**6.5**	**5.5**
Bigger States									
1. Andhra Pradesh	7.3	7.7	6.9	7.9	8.4	7.4	5.9	6.1	5.7
2. Assam	8.7	9.3	7.9	9.2	9.8	8.5	5.6	6.6	4.6
3. Bihar	8.1	8.2	8.0	8.3	8.4	8.1	6.6	6.5	6.7
4. Chhattisgarh	8.1	8.6	7.6	8.4	8.7	8.0	6.9	8.2	5.6
5. Delhi	4.6	4.7	4.6	5.5	6.0	4.9	4.5	4.5	4.5
6. Gujarat	7.1	7.6	6.6	8.0	8.8	7.2	5.8	5.9	5.7
7. Haryana	6.7	7.0	6.3	7.0	7.4	6.5	5.8	5.8	5.8
8. Jammu & Kashmir	5.5	5.8	5.3	5.7	5.8	5.5	5.0	5.8	4.3
9. Jharkhand	7.9	7.9	7.8	8.4	8.3	8.5	5.7	6.4	4.9
10. Karnataka	7.1	7.6	6.6	7.9	8.3	7.5	5.6	6.3	4.9
11. Kerala	6.4	7.6	5.2	6.3	7.6	5.2	6.5	7.8	5.3
12. Madhya Pradesh	9.0	9.2	8.6	9.8	10.1	9.5	6.1	6.4	5.7
13. Maharashtra	6.7	7.4	5.9	7.4	8.3	6.5	5.7	6.2	5.1

1	2	3	4	5	6	7	8	9	10
14. Orissa	9.5	10.1	8.8	9.9	10.5	9.2	7.0	7.2	6.8
15. Punjab	6.7	7.2	6.1	7.2	7.8	6.6	5.8	6.2	5.4
16. Rajasthan	7.0	7.0	6.9	7.2	7.2	7.2	6.2	6.5	5.9
17. Tamil Nadu	7.4	8.0	6.7	8.2	8.7	7.6	6.2	7.1	5.4
18. Uttar Pradesh	8.7	8.8	8.6	9.1	9.2	9.1	6.8	7.0	6.5
19. West Bengal	6.4	7.0	5.7	6.3	6.8	5.7	6.6	7.5	5.6
Smaller States									
1. Arunachal Pradesh	5.0	5.3	4.6	5.5	5.8	5.2	2.8	3.3	2.3
2. Goa	7.1	8.1	6.1	8.9	9.9	8.0	5.8	6.8	4.9
3. Himachal Pradesh	6.9	7.6	6.1	7.1	7.9	6.4	4.7	5.3	4.0
4. Manipur	4.1	4.7	3.5	4.0	4.4	3.5	4.4	5.5	3.3
5. Meghalaya	7.5	8.9	6.2	7.9	9.1	6.7	6.0	8.3	3.7
6. Mizoram	5.1	6.0	4.2	6.2	6.7	5.6	4.1	5.3	2.9
7. Nagaland	3.8	4.4	3.2	4.0	4.8	3.1	3.1	2.6	3.7
8. Sikkim	5.1	5.7	4.5	5.2	5.6	4.7	4.8	6.2	3.3
9. Tripura	5.7	6.6	4.9	5.7	6.5	4.9	5.8	7.2	4.5
10. Uttaranchal	7.4	8.0	6.6	7.9	8.9	6.9	5.3	5.2	5.5

1	2	3	4	5	6	7	8	9	10
Union Territories									
1. Andaman & Nicobar Islands	4.7	5.3	3.9	5.3	5.6	5.0	3.6	4.9	2.1
2. Chandigarh	4.5	5.3	3.6	2.7	3.1	2.0	4.7	5.5	3.8
3. Dadra & Nagar Haveli	5.1	4.7	5.6	5.6	5.4	5.9	3.1	2.2	4.4
4. Daman & Diu	5.6	6.8	4.2	5.3	6.1	4.3	6.1	7.9	4.0
5. Lakshadweep	6.3	6.7	6.0	7.5	7.4	7.6	5.2	6.0	4.4
6. Pondicherry	7.1	8.7	5.6	8.0	9.5	6.4	6.7	8.2	5.2

Table 4. Infant mortality rate by sex and residence, 2005

India/States/ Union Territories	Total			Rural			Urban		
	Total	Male	Female	Total	Male	Female	Total	Male	Female
1	2	3	4	5	6	7	8	9	10
India	**58**	**56**	**61**	**64**	**62**	**66**	**40**	**37**	**43**
Bigger States									
1. Andhra Pradesh	57	56	58	63	62	64	39	38	40
2. Assam	68	66	69	71	69	72	39	36	43
3. Bihar	61	60	62	62	61	63	47	45	50
4. Chhattisgarh	63	63	64	65	65	66	52	49	55
5. Delhi	35	33	37	44	50	36	33	30	37
6. Gujarat	54	52	55	63	61	64	37	36	38
7. Haryana	60	51	70	64	55	76	45	40	52
8. Jammu & Kashmir	50	47	55	53	49	58	39	36	43
9. Jharkhand	50	43	58	53	45	62	33	31	35
10. Karnataka	50	48	51	54	54	55	39	37	42
11. Kerala	14	14	15	15	15	16	12	11	14
12. Madhya Pradesh	76	72	79	80	77	84	54	52	56
13. Maharashtra	36	34	37	41	40	42	27	25	29

	1	*2*	*3*	*4*	*5*	*6*	*7*	*8*	*9*	*10*
14.	Orissa	75	74	77	78	77	79	55	50	61
15.	Punjab	44	41	48	49	46	51	37	32	43
16.	Rajasthan	68	64	72	75	71	79	43	37	49
17.	Tamil Nadu	37	35	39	39	38	40	34	30	39
18.	Uttar Pradesh	73	71	75	77	75	79	54	53	55
19.	West Bengal	38	38	39	40	40	40	31	28	35
Smaller States										
1.	Arunachal Pradesh	37	29	46						
2.	Goa	16	14	17						
3.	Himachal Pradesh	49	47	51						
4.	Manipur	13	12	13						
5.	Meghalaya	49	48	51						
6.	Mizoram	20	18	22						
7.	Nagaland	18	19	18						
8.	Sikkim	30	29	31						
9.	Tripura	31	30	31						
10.	Uttaranchal	42	37	48						

Infant mortality rates for smaller States and Union Territories are based on three-years period 2003-05. On account of wide year-to-year fluctuations due to inadequate sample size, the infant mortality rate by sex, separately for rural and urban areas is not given.

1	2	3	4	5	6	7	8	9	10
Union Territories									
1. Andaman & Nicobar Islands	27	26	27						
2. Chandigarh	19	17	22						
3. Dadra & Nagar Haveli	42	42	43						
4. Daman & Diu	28	27	28						
5. Lakshadweep	22	23	21						
6. Pondicherry	28	29	27						

ABOUT THE SAMPLE REGISTRATION SYSTEM (SRS)

The Sample Registration System (SRS) is a large-scale demographic survey for providing reliable annual estimates of birth rate, death rate and other fertility & mortality indicators at the national and sub-national levels. Initiated on a pilot basis by the OFFICE OF THE REGISTRAR GENERAL, INDIA in a few selected states in 1964-65, it became fully operational during 1969-70 with about 3700 sample units. The field investigation consists of continuous enumeration of births and deaths in selected sample units by resident part time enumerators, generally anganwadi workers & teachers, and an independent survey every six months by SRS supervisors. The data obtained by these two independent functionaries are matched. The unmatched and partially matched events are re-verified in the field and thereafter an unduplicated count of births and deaths is obtained. The sample unit in rural areas is a village or a segment of it, if the village population is 2000 or more. In urban areas, the sampling unit is a census enumeration block with population ranging from 750 to 1000. The SRS sample is replaced every ten years based on the latest census frame. It had been a practice to stagger the replacement process over 2-3 years. However, the latest replacement has been carried out in one go. Effective from January 2004, this sample is based on the 2001 Census frame. At present, SRS is operational in 7,597 sample units (4,433 rural and 3,164 urban) spread across all States and Union territories and covers about 1.3 million households and 6.83 million population.

Number of sample units and population covered, India, States and Union Territories, 2005

India/States/ Union Territories	*Number of sample units*			*Population covered (in '000)*		
	Total	*Rural*	*Urban*	*Total*	*Rural*	*Urban*
1	*2*	*3*	*4*	*5*	*6*	*7*
India	**7,597**	**4,433**	**3,164**	**6,830**	**3,513**	**3,318**
Bigger States						
1. Andhra Pradesh	375	235	140	394	199	195
2. Assam	300	90	210	195	101	94

1	*2*	*3*	*4*	*5*	*6*	*7*
3. Bihar	330	200	130	334	175	159
4. Chhattisgarh	130	40	90	99	51	48
5. Delhi	200	10	190	142	77	65
6. Gujarat	365	215	150	351	181	170
7. Haryana	210	100	110	202	108	94
8. Jammu & Kashmir	260	150	110	213	111	102
9. Jharkhand	170	60	110	112	59	53
10. Karnataka	480	330	150	431	216	215
11. Kerala	250	150	100	333	161	172
12. Madhya Pradesh	340	220	120	305	159	146
13. Maharashtra	485	250	235	398	204	194
14. Orissa	405	290	115	324	163	161
15. Punjab	250	150	100	235	124	111
16. Rajasthan	350	250	100	317	166	151
17. Tamil Nadu	465	250	215	448	225	223
18. Uttar Pradesh	500	350	150	537	284	253
19. West Bengal	555	310	245	555	286	269

1	2	3	4	5	6	7
Smaller States						
1. Arunachal Pradesh	60	45	15	30	16	15
2. Goa	85	43	42	76	38	38
3. Himachal Pradesh	190	140	50	92	46	46
4. Manipur	150	110	40	129	65	64
5. Meghalaya	120	90	30	61	30	30
6. Mizoram	40	20	20	29	15	15
7. Nagaland	45	33	12	36	19	17
8. Sikkim	60	45	15	57	29	27
9. Tripura	80	60	20	102	52	50
10. Uttaranchal	150	100	50	108	56	52
Union Territories						
1. Andaman & Nicobar Islands	50	34	16	33	17	16
2. Chandigarh	35	5	30	30	17	13
3. Dadra & Nagar Haveli	30	22	8	37	20	17
4. Daman & Diu	20	13	7	26	15	12
5. Lakshadweep	12	6	6	14	7	7
6. Pondicherry	50	17	33	44	22	22

Note: 1. Population figures exclude that of 3 rural units of West Bengal, 1 urban unit of Jharkhand, 2 rural units of Chhattisgarh, 1 rural unit of Maharashtra, and 4 rural units of Andaman & Nicobar Islands due to non-receipt of returns.

2. 'Total' population may not add up to 'Rural' and 'Urban' population due to rounding.

Statement 2

Expectation of life at age 1 by sex and residence, India

Mid year	*Total*			*Rural*			*Urban*		
	Total	*Male*	*Female*	*Total*	*Male*	*Female*	*Total*	*Male*	*Female*
2001	66.3	65.3	67.2	65.4	64.3	66.1	70.2	68.6	71.5
2002	66.5	65.5	67.4	65.5	64.5	66.2	70.3	68.6	71.7

Statement 5 / **Statement 6** / **Statement 7**

India & States	**Total**		**Male** *Expectation of life at age*		**Female** *Expectation of life at age*	
	Life expectancy at birth	*Life expectancy at age 1*	*Life expectancy at birth*	*Life expectancy at age 1*	*Life expectancy at birth*	*Life expectancy at age 1*
India **2002**	63.0	66.5	62.1	65.5	63.7	67.4
Andhra Pradesh	63.9	7.2	62.4	65.7	65.0	68.3
Assam	58.3	62.4	58.0	62.0	58.6	62.7
Bihar	61.2	64.1	61.8	64.7	59.9	62.9
Gujarat	63.7	66.9	62.7	65.6	64.8	68.2
Haryana	65.6	69.6	65.3	68.9	66.8	68.9
Himachal Pradesh	66.5	69.0	66.1	68.9	66.8	68.9

Karnataka	64.9	67.9	63.1	66.2	66.7	69.5
Kerala	73.7	73.5	71.0	70.8	76.1	75.9
Madhya Pradesh	57.4	62.4	57.5	62.3	57.2	62.5
Maharashtra	66.6	68.7	65.5	67.4	67.8	70.1
Orissa	58.9	63.3	58.9	63.5	58.9	63.1
Punjab	68.9	71.9	67.8	70.2	69.8	73.7
Rajasthan	61.5	66.3	60.9	65.5	62.0	67.1
Tamil Nadu	65.7	67.8	64.6	66.6	66.8	68.9
Uttar Pradesh	59.6	64.2	59.9	64.4	59.0	63.9
West Bengal	64.4	66.7	63.7	66.2	65.2	67.4

Source : SRS Statistical Report 2003
Indicator : Early neonatal deaths as percentage of infant deaths

	2003			*2004*			*2005*		
	Total	*Rural*	*Urban*	*Total*	*Rural*	*Urban*	*Total*	*Rural*	*Urban*
India	**40.9**	**42.2**	**31.4**	**64.1**	**64.9**	**59.7**	**62.9**	**63.7**	**58.2**
Andhra Pradesh	35.8	37.9	20.8	60.8	64.2	42.8	61.1	68	28.7
Assam	34	34	33.8	52.5	52.2	58.5	49.2	49.4	45.5
Bihar	32.4	32.1	36.9	53.8	54.6	42.6	53.1	54.2	37.5
Chhattisgarh				71.8	70.8	79.4	70.3	70.5	68.5

	2003			2004			2005		
	Total	*Rural*	*Urban*	*Total*	*Rural*	*Urban*	*Total*	*Rural*	*Urban*
Delhi				62.6	37.9	69.6	57.5	38	62
Gujarat	42.3	39.4	56.9	68.8	67.4	73	66.3	63.9	74.1
Haryana	28.7	29.6	23.5	51.4	49.7	58.6	58.7	58.3	60.3
Himachal Pradesh	57.6	57.8	49.3	59.3	58.9	79.8	62.4	62.9	50
Jammu & Kashmir				77.5	77.4	78.6	71.6	70.4	80.3
Jharkhand				52.9	54.4	39.3	56.2	57	48.3
Karnataka	40.2	40.1	41.2	51.2	57.4	30.7	56.9	62.8	38.1
Kerala	40.9	39	48.7	75	75	75.3	75.9	74.3	81.9
Madhya Pradesh	40.7	40.6	41.2	62.8	63	61.7	67	67.1	66.8
Maharashtra	44.3	47	37.1	72.9	75.5	66.7	70.8	71.9	68.3
Orissa	42.3	42.9	33.2	63	63.2	60.9	70.6	71.6	58.7
Punjab	37.1	39.5	24.1	66.4	67.8	63.1	67.3	68.9	63.5
Rajasthan	43.8	44.5	36.9	62.4	60.5	75.5	63	63.7	58.8
Tamil Nadu	48.9	49.6	46.3	71.5	78.8	57.7	70.9	80.7	54.9
Uttar Pradesh	42.6	44.8	23.7	69.7	70.9	61.6	61.6	61.7	61.4
West Bengal	47.3	51.4	19.4	72.5	75.9	53.2	76.8	79.1	64

Statement 1

Expectation of life at birth by sex and residence, India

Mid year	*Total*			*Rural*			*Urban*		
	Total	*Male*	*Female*	*Total*	*Male*	*Female*	*Total*	*Male*	*Female*
2001	62.7	61.8	63.5	61.4	60.5	62.0	68.1	66.5	69.4
2002	63.0	62.1	63.7	61.6	60.8	62.2	68.3	66.7	69.6

Source: As mentioned below Indicator: Maternal Mortality Ratio

	1997-1998	*1999-2001*	*2001-2003*
INDIA TOTAL	**398**	**327**	**301**
Andhra Pradesh	197	220	195
Assam	568	398	490
Bihar/Jharkhand	531	400	371
Gujarat	46	202	172
Haryana	136	176	162
Karnataka	245	266	228
Kerala	150	149	110
Madhya Pradesh	441	407	379
Maharashtra	166	169	149

	1997-1998	1999-2001	2001-2003
Orissa	346	424	358
Punjab	280	177	178
Rajasthan	508	501	445
Tamil Nadu	131	167	134
Uttar Pradesh	606	539	517
West Bengal	303	218	194

* Includes others
1997-98 source: SRS Special Maternal Mortality; Special Fertility & Motarlity Survey
1999-2001 source: SRS Prospective Household Reports
2001-2003 source: SRS Special Survey of Deaths

Indicator		*Latest available data*	*Year*	*Source*	*Remarks*
Manufacturing (*a*) {food beverage, textiles, wood, paper, leather}					
	Urban	26.1	1993-94	16	
	Rural	37.0	1993-94	16	
Manufacturing (*b*) {chemicals except petrol non-metallic minerals, basic metals, metals and machinery, transport equipment parts, and others}					
	Urban	11.8	1993-94	16	
	Rural	19.7	1993-94	16	
Electricity, gas and water					
	Urban	3.7	1993-94	16	
	Rural	4.5	1993-94	16	
Construction	Urban	14.1	1993-94	16	
	Rural	11.3	1993-94	16	
Women as a per cent of all Employers[m]	Urban	13.80	1993-94	16	
	Rural	17.20	1993-94	16	
Unpaid family workers	Urban	39.24	1993-94	16	
	Rural	58.50	1993-94	16	
Own account workers		14.57	1993-94	16	
Employees"		15.64	1993-94	16	
Unemployed women as a per cent of total unemployed population		46.52	1993-94	18	
Women and Education					
Literacy rate (%)					
	Total	39.29°	1991	11	
Female	15-24 years	49.35°	1991	11	
	25+ years	27.80°	1991	11	
	Total	64.13°	1991	11	

Indicator		*Latest available data*	*Year*	*Source*	*Remarks*
Male	15-24 years	73.50°	1991	11	
	25+ years	57.10°	1991	11	
Mean years of schooling					
	Total	2.4	1992	19	
	Female	1.2	1992	19	
	Male	3.5	1992	19	
Health Resources					
Per capita health expenditure (US $)		17	1993	11	
Government health expenditure as a per cent of total expenditure		3.47	1993-94	12	
Average daily caloric supply per capita					
Urban		2259	1997-98	13	Relates to
Rural		2321	1997-98	13	18 states
Daily per capita caloric supply as a per cent of the recommended daily allowance: Urban		93.2	1998	14	
Rural		97.7	1998	13	
Women as a per cent of total physicians[9]		22.61	1995	15	
2. WOMEN'S STATUS					
Women and Work					
Economically active female population 15 years and above (% of total female .population in the same age group)					
Urban		18.45	1993-94	16	
Rural		37.91	1993-94	16	

Indicator	*Latest available data*	*Year*	*Source*	*Remarks*
Economically active female children (% of all female children in the 10-14 age group) Urban	4.70	1993-94	16	
Rural	14.20	1993-94	16	
Women as a per cent of all workers in the				
Organized sector[h]	15.8	1996	17	
Unorganized sector[i]	33.9	1993-94	16	
Employed women as a per cent of total employed population by sector Agriculture				
Principal status[i] Urban	31.6	1993-94	16	
Rural	31.5	1993-94	16	
Services[k]				
Principal status[j] Urban	29.6	1993-94	16	
Rural	21.6	1993-94	16	
Services (b)[l]				
Principal status[j] Urban	12.4	1993-94	16	
Rural	8.1	1993-94	16	
Industry—Principal status[i]				
Mining and quarrying Urban	11.0	1993-94	16	
Rural	22.0	1993-94	16	
General fertility rate (per 1000 women of reproductive age) Total	117.0	1995	22	
Urban	87.3	1995	22	
Rural	126.7	1995	22	
Total fertility rate (15-49 years)				
Total	3.5	1995	22	
Urban	2.6	1995	22	
Rural	3.9	1995	22	

Indicator		*Latest available data*	*Year*	*Source*	*Remarks*
Fertility rate of women 15-19 years (per 1000 women of the same age group)		55.2	1995	22	
Sex differentials in children's health and nutritional status					
Infant mortality rate (per 1000 live births)	Female	72.2°	1997	23	
	Male	70.3°	1997	23	
Child mortality rate (per 1000 population in the 1-4 year age group)	Female	42.0	1992-3	7	Data pertain to the period tengear preceding the sur- vey
	Male	29.4	192-93	7	
Children (12-23 months) fully immunized against EPI-target diseases[r]	Total	48.5	1994	24	
	Female	47.5	1994	24	
	Male	48.5	1994	24	
Children under five years who are underweight (% with low weight-for-age)					
Urban	Female	45.3	1998	13	
	Male	43.6	1998	13	
Rural	Female	50.0	1998	13	
	Male	50.2	1998	13	
Children under five years who are stunted (% with low height-for-age)					
Urban	Female	50.2	1998	13	
	Male	51.9	1998	13	
Rural	Female	57.2	1998	13	
	Male	58.0	1998	13	

Indicator		*Latest available data*	*Year*	*Source*	*Remarks*
Children under five years who are wasted (% with low weight-for-height)					
Urban	Female	27.6	1998	13	
	Male	15.1	1998	13	
Rural	Female	24.0	1998	13	
	Male	16.0	1998	13	
Primary school net enrolment (%)					
Urban	Female	70.20	1991	11	
	Male	74.70	1991	11	
Rural	Female	42.50	1991	11	
	Male	53.20	1991	11	
Secondary school net enrolment[q] (%)					
Urban	Female	80.68	1991	11	
	Male	86.57	1991	11	
Rural	Female	57.57	1991	11	
	Male	76.80	1991	11	
Female enrolment in higher secondary school (% of total)		35.28	1995-96	19	
Female enrolment in vocational/ technical institutions (% of total)		3.31	1990-91	19	
Female enrolment in university and professional courses (% of total)		33.20	1993-94	5	
Women as a per cent of total school teachers	Primary	37.78	1995-96	19	
	Secondary	35.11	1995-96	19	
Women's participation in political and public decision-making					
Parliament seats occupied by women (%)					
	Lower House	7.95	1998	20	
	Upper House	8.6	1996	20	
Ministerial positions held by women (%)		9.5	1998	20	
Sub-ministerial positions held by women (%)					
All India and central services		8.4	1995-96	5	
Women judges in supreme/high courts		3.0	1996	21	

Indicator		*Latest available data*	*Year*	*Source*	*Remarks*
3. WOMEN'S HEALTH STATUS					
Demographic indicators					
Sex ratio (males per 100 females)					
	At birth	112°	1991-93	22	
In general population					
	Total	108[a]	1991	1	
	Urban	107.87[a]	1991	1	
	Rural	106.60[a]	1991	1	
Life expectancy at birth (years)					
	Total	60.3°	1991-95	22	
	Female	60.9°	1191-95	22	
	Male	59.7°	1991-5	22	
Per cent of women					
15-19 years currently married		2.6°	1995	22	
20-59 years currently married		41.1°	1995	22	
60 years and above currently married		2.9°	1995	22	
Women's health status					
Anaemia prevalence in pregnant women 15-49 years (%			87.5	1991	12
Number of women diagnosed with AIDS		1177	1998	25	
Maternal mortality ratio (per 100,000 live births)	Total	420	1992-93	7	
	15-19 year olds	965	1986-90	26	
Abortion rate (per 1000 live births)		452[a]	1994	27	Estimate
Perinatal mortality rate (per 1000 total births)		42.5	1994	28	
Birth weight less than 2500 grams (%)		31	1991-93	12	
Contraceptive prevalence rate (%)					
Total		40.6	1992-193	7	
By method	Pill	1.2	1992-93	7	
	IUD	1.9	1992-93	7	

Indicator	*Latest available data*	*Year*	*Source*	*Remarks*
Injections	0.1	1992-93	7	
Condoms	2.4	1992-93	7	
Female sterilization	27.3	1992-93	7	
Male sterilization	3.4	1992-93	7	
Periodic abstinence	2.6	1992-93	7	
Withdrawal	1.4	1992-93	7	
Other methods	0.2	1992-93	7	
Not using any methods	59.4	1992-93	7	
Pregnant women attended by trained personnel[t] (%)	49.1	1992-93	7	Data pertain to the four years preced ing the survey
Pregnant women immunized with two or more doses of tetanus toxoid (%)	53.8	1992-93	7	
Deliveries attended by trained personnel" (%)	34.2	1992-93	7	
Deliveries occurring in public and private health facilities	24.5	1992-93	7	
Health risks related to lifestyle and environment				
Population with access to safe drinking water (%) Total	81	1990-96	2	
Urban	85	1990-96	2	
Rural	79	1990-96	2	
Population with access to sanitation facilities (%) Total	29	1990-96	2	
Urban	70	1990-96	2	
Rural	14	1990-96	2	
Annual rate of deforestation (%)	0.6	1981-90	29	
Water withdrawal per annum as a per cent of available resources	18	1980-89	29	
Estimated number of rural women affected by scarcity of firewood (in thousands)	172,140	1990	30	

Notes

[a] Includes population projection for Jammu and Kashmir where 1991 census was not held.

[b] Includes currently married, widowed, divorced, separated.

[c] Relates to those married among females.

[d] Includes agriculture, forestry and logging, fishery, mining, and quarrying.

[e] Poverty line based on expenditure required for purchasing food, consumption of which would ensure 2100 k.cal. for those in urban areas and 2400 k.cal. for those in rural areas.

[f] Defence expenditure is taken from the revised budget estimate of Ministry of Finance.

[g] Relates to number of graduates registered with state medical councils as of 31 December of the respective year.

[h] Includes all the establishments in the public sector and non-organizational agricultural establishments employing or more persons in the private sector.

[i] Derived by subtracting the organized sector figures from the total work force figures of all sectors.

[j] A person, who pursued for a relatively longer time during the preceding one year, one or more economic activities is considered as "principally" working or employed in a given sector.

[k] Includes community, social and personal services.

[l] Includes financing, insurance, and real estate and business services.

[m] Includes own account workers and is based on figures from *Structural changes in women's employment.*

[n] Includes regular salaried and wage employees and is estimated based on figures from *Structural changes in women's employment.*

[o] Excludes Jammu and Kashmir.

[p] Enrolment calculated by looking at the school going children at the age of 7 to the single age returned at 7 in the census.

[q] Enrolment calculated by looking at the school going children at the age of 11 to the single age returned at in the census.

[r] EPI-target diseases include diptheria, whooping cough, tetanus, polio, tuberculosis and measles.

[s] Includes spontaneous and induced abortions.

[t] Relates to antenatal care provided by doctors and other health professionals outside the home.

[u] Trained personnel includes doctor and nurse/midwife.

Sources[1]

1. Office of the Registrar-General, India. *Census of India 1991.* New Delhi; 1992.
2. United Nations Population Fund, *The state of world population 1998,* New York; 1998.
3. United Nations. *Demographic yearbook 1997.* New York: United Nations; 1998.
4. National Sample Survey Organization, Department of Statistics. *Sarvekshana 1990.* New Delhi; 1990.
5. Office of the Registrar-General, India. *Women in India: a statistical profile.* New Delhi; 1997.
6. World Health Organization, *The world health report 1998.* Geneva; 1998.
7. International Institute for Population Sciences. *National family health survey (MCH and Family Planning). India 1992-93.* Mumbai (Bombay) : UPS; 1995.
8. Central Statistical Organisation, Department of Statistics, Ministry of Planning and Programme Implementation. *Women and men in India, 1995.* New Delhi; 1995.
9. United Nations. *Human development report 1999.* New York: Oxford University Press; 1999.
10. Economic Division, Ministry of Finance. *Economic Survey 1998.* New Delhi; 1998.
11. Sundar R. *Household survey of health care utilisation and expenditure.* Working paper no. 53. New Delhi: National Council for Applied Economics Research; 1995.

---

1. Data from Indian nutrition profile 1998, Department of Women and Child Development, Ministry of Human Resource Development, New Delhi.

12. Ministry of Health and Family Welfare. *India country report on the third evaluation of the implementation of the health for all strategy.* New Delhi; 1997.

13. Data from Indian nutrition profile 1998, Department of Women and Child Development, Ministry of Human Resource Development, New Delhi.

14. Data from National Nutrition Monitoring Bureau, National Institute of Nutrition, Indian Council for Medical Research, Hyderabad, India; 1998.

15. Data from Indian Medical Council, New Delhi.

16. National Sample Survey Organisation, Department of Statistics. *Sarvekshana 50th round report: structural changes in women's employment.* New Delhi; 1998.

17. Data from manpower profile India, 1997, Institute of Applied Manpower Research, New Delhi.

18. Data from Annual Report of the Ministry of Labour, 1996-97, New Delhi.

19. Data from Department of Education, Ministry of Human Resource Development, New Delhi; 1991.

20. Data from Lok Sabha Secretariat cited in Central Statistical Organisation, Department of Statistics, Ministry of Planning and Programme Implementation. *Women and Men in India, 1998.* New Delhi; 1998.

21. Data from Department of Justice, Ministry of Law and Justice cited in Central Statistical Organisation, Department of Statistics, Ministry of Planning and Programme Implementation. *Women and Men in India, 1998.* New Delhi; 1998.

22. Data from Registrar-General, India. Sample registration system cited in Central Statistical Organisation, Department of Statistics, Ministry of Planning and Programme Implementation. *Women and Men in India,* 1998. New Delhi; 1998.

23. Registrar-General, India. *SRS bulletin,* Vol. 33, No.1, 1999 April, New Delhi; 1999.

24. Data from National Council of Applied Economic Research cited in UNICEF. *Rights and opportunities: situation of*

children and women in India. New York: Oxford University Press; 1997.

25. Data from Annual Report of Ministry of Health and Family Welfare, New Delhi; 1998.
26. Data from National Institute of Public Cooperation and Child Development. *Statistics on children and women in India 1997,* New Delhi; 1997.
27. Chabra R. et al. *Abortion in India.* New Delhi; 1994.
28. Data from Registrar-General, India. Sample registration system cited in UNICEF. *Rights and opportunities, situation of children and women in India.* New York; 1997.
29. Haq M. *Human development in South Asia.* Karachi: Human Development Center and Oxford University Press; 1997.
30. United Nations. *The world's women 1995: trends and statistics.* New York: United Nations; 1995.

---

1. Data from sources 1, 4-5, 8, 10-19, 24-29 are as cited in Gopalan S. Shiva M. editors. *National profile on women, health and development: India.* New Delhi: Voluntary Health Association of India; 1999.

F. No. O 15012/7/2006–SSR
Government of India
Planning Commission
(SER Division)

Yojana Bhavan, Sansad Marg
New Delhi – 110 001
Dated : 28th July, 2008

To,

The Executive Director.
Indian Trust for Innovation and Social Change.
ITISC, EB,/166, Maya Enclave,
New Delhi - 110 064

Subject: Publication of study Report titled "**Socio Economic Causes and Determinants Behind Infant Mortality Rate (IMR) & Maternal Mortality Rate (MMR)**" -

Madam,

I am directed to refer to your letter number dated 15th July, 2008 requesting for publication of the above study report. The permission to publish the findings of the report is hereby accorded, subject to the acceptance of the following conditions:

1. Ten copies of the publised *version of the report* will have to be submitted to the Planning Commission.

2. You will clearly acknowledge that the present publication is the outcome of the Study on the subject cited above.

3. ***Planning Commission is not responsible for findings of or opinions expressed in a document prepared with the support provided under the SER Scheme. This responsibility vests with the Researcher/***

Institution that received the grants-in-aid under the Scheme.

4. The fact that Planning Commission provided financial support under the Scheme of SER will be acknowledged on any document produced with its support, whether or not circulated widely, and the **Disclaimer at Sr. No. 3** above will be prominently displayed on such a document.

Yours Faithfully

(S. Mukherjee)

Deputy Secretary to the GOI

Ph. 23096791

BIBLIOGRAPHY

LITERATURE CONSULTED

1. Improving Women's Health in India (World Bank Publication) (Series Development in Practice-Washington DC, 1996).
2. Pre-birth elimination of females. (A handbook of guidelines - Centre for Women's Development Studies).
3. Report No. 3 of 2004 (Office of the Registrar General, India, Man Singh Road, New Delhi).
4. (World Bank) Indian Women - Their Health and Economic Productivity, Meera Chatterjee (WDP-109).
5. Medical Certification of Cause of Death -1998 (Office of the Registrar General - India - Ministry of Home Affairs - New Delhi).
6. National Rural Health Mission (2005-2012) Mission Document.
7. Ministry of Health and Family Welfare NRHM (Action Points).
8. Child Mortality in Rural India (Bas Van der Klaavw—Limin Wang - April 2004).
9. Annual Report (1982-83) Ministry of Health and Family Welfare, New Delhi.
10. Annual Report (1993-1994) Ministry of Health and Family Welfare, Government of India.
11. Perinatal and New Born Care in Pakistan (extracts). Early Child Health and Survival in Pakistan.
12. Reduction of Infant Mortality and Trends in Infant Mortality.
13. National Library of Medicine - Impact of Development and Population Policies on Fertility in India, Jain, A.K.

14. World Health Organisation, (Regional Office for South East Asia (Maternal, new born and Child Health situation in India).
15. Reproductive and Child Health Project (May 27, 2005) (Document of the World Bank).
16. Age Specific Death Rates in India -1988.
17. The second integrated child development Services Project (ICDS).
18. Child labour, nutrition and Education in Rural India (Alessandro Cigno Furio Camillo Rosati, Zafiris Tzannatos.
19. Diet and Nutrition - a holistic approach - Rudolph Ballentine, M.D.
20. Reaching out to the Child (South Asia Education Sector Working Paper No. 1).
21. "Derlp" essential to reduce infant mortality rate in India - experience from Ballabhgarh Project.
22. Infant and Child Mortality in India. A comparative study in 3 selected States. (Sangha Mitro Panda 25th April 2005) Guide Prof. Subrata Lahiri.
23. India: Issues in Women's Health. January 25, 1996 - (South Asia Country Department II).
24. Sample Registration System - SRS Bulletin. (Estimated Infrant Mortality Rate -1998 (Provisional) 1998.
25. April 1999 SRS Bulletin.
26. SRS Bulletin 2000/October 2000.
27. SRS Bulletin 2001.
28. SRS Bulletin October, 2002.
29. SRS Bulletin 2003.
30. SRS Bulletin - April, 2004.
31. SRS Bulletin April, 2005.

32. SRS Bulletin April, 2006.
33. NIAHRD study of social factors contributing to Maternal Mortality - Orissa State Report.
34. Poverty, Class and Health Culture in India Debabar Banerji - Prachi Prakashan, New Delhi.
35. Transnatural Curing Page (236). David G. Mandelbaum.
36. Folk medicine in a North Indian Village R.S. Khare (266-285).
37. A North Indian Healer and the sources of his Power - Edward O. Henry (286-307).
38. Traditional Health Practices of Kumaoni Women. Continuity and Change Anjali Capila, Reader Lady Irwin College, University of Delhi 2004 (Concept Publishing Co., New Delhi-110059.
39. Infant Mortality in India edt. by Anirudh K. Jain and Pravin Visaria (Gujarat Institute of Area Planning, Ahmedabad).
40. Level Trends and Determinants of Infant Mortality in Rural India - Seela Visaria.
41. Impact of RUHA's Health and Development Program on Infant Mortality - Rajaratnan Abel.
42. Community based studies on Infant Mortality in Haryana, Vijay Kumar and Neena Dutta.
43. Correlates of Infant Survival according to Cohort Study in Vadu Rural Health Project, V.N. Rao and Banoo Coyaji.
44. Evidence from selected states Infant Mortality in Uttar Pradesh, M.E. Khan.
45. Correlates of Infant Mortality in Madurai Dt. of Tamil Nadu, S. Gunasekaran.

46. Correlates of Infant Mortality in Rural Area of Tamil Nadu, C. Ramanujam.
47. Infant Mortality - an analysis of Recent Births in Gujarat - M.M. Gandotra and Narayan Das.
48. Factors associated with Infant Mortality in Rajasthan and Orissa - Tara Kanitkar and B.N. Murthy.
49. Infant Mortality - some evidence from Rural Madhya Pradesh.
50. Some Issues in the Selection and Assessment of the Determinants of Infant Mortality, K. Srinivasan.
51. A framework for the Study of Proximate Determinants of Infant Mortality in Less Developed Countries : Moninag.
52. World Development Indicators - 2000.
53. Choose the Sex of Your Child, Dr. Inderjit Kaur Barthakur.
54. The endangered Sex - Barbara D. Miller.
55. The Wrongs of Indian Womanhood Mrs. Marcus B. Fuller, Oliphant Andersan and Ferrier 1900.
56. Health and Disease. An epidemological Background, Kingsley Davis - World Urbanism (1950-1970).
57. Effect of gender of Head of Household on Women's and Children's nutritional status, Eileen Kennedy, Pauline Peters and Lawrence Haddad.
58. Number of Recognised Training Centres for different courses -1990.
59. India the next 7000 Days - Dr. Satish C. Seth (Wiley Eastern 1985).
60. From Shadows to self India Women's Watch NGO Country Report Beijing + 10 Review (2005).
61. UGC Workshop on Capacity Building for Women Managers in Higher Education - Centre for Women's Studies and Development, BHU.

62. Task force on Women empowerment, Government of Karnataka (2001).

63. The Paradigm of Contradiction. The eclipsed Woman in Theories of (2002) BHU. Democracy - Centre for Women's Studies and Development.

64. Looking at Woman : Reevaluation of some of the ancient Indian texts - Chandrakala Padia BHU Centre for Women's Studies and Development.

65. Globalisation, Politics and Women U. Kalpagam, BHU Centre for Women's Studies and Development, 2003.

66. Reaching out to the Child An Integrated Approach to Child Development - The World Bank (Human Development Sector South Asia Region - September, 2004.

67. Mapping India's Children - Unicef in action 2004-2005.

68. The Social Science Encyclopaedia Edited by Adam Kuper and Jessica Kuper - Routledge and Kegan Paul (London, Boston and Henley).

69. Superstition, Human Rights and Imperatives of Future (ITISC 2004).

70. Five Year Plans - Three volumes (2002-2007) Vol. I, Vol. II and Vol. III.

71. Midterm appraisal of the Tenth Five Year Plan.

72. Sacred Rites and Ceremonies (Encyclopedia Britannica - Vol. 26, Pages 770-839.

73. Seventh Women's Global Leadership Institute - Challenges of the New Millennium, June 7-18, 1999.

74. We need a War against female foeticide - Dr. Sharda Jain, President East Delhi Gynecologist Forum.

75. Managing Development for Future - A Study in Transition - Satish C. Seth (Gyan 2001) Vol. I and II.

76. 10th Plan strategies for children (Govt. of India).

77. India's Five Year Plans complete documents, 1951-56 to 2002-2007 (Mid term appraisal) June 28, 2005 (Academic Foundation) New Delhi (Jain Book Agency).
78. Indian Ritual and Belief - The Keys of Power J. Abbott B.A. (Oxon) 1932, ICS, Usha Publications 1984, Daryaganj, Delhi.
79. Faiths, Fares and Festivals of India, C.H. Buck - (398-38 IIC), Rupa Hoj.
80. Attitude assessment of male adolescents in Ratanpur and Laxmipur Blocks of Maharajganj district of Uttar Pradesh.
81. Maternal Death Investigations Purulia, West Bengal - 2005.
82. Sample Registration System - Maternal Mortality in India -1997-2003, Trends, Causes and Risk factors.
83. Journal of Women's Health (An analysis of the Determinants of Maternal Mortality in Sub-Saharan Africa) October 2004.
84. Challenges to Women's Reproductive Health - Maternal Mortality - Zoe Oxaal with Sally Baden (September 1996 - revised October1996).
85. Determinants of Maternal Care in a Region of South India - Jagdish C. Bhatia and John Cleland (Institute of Management - Bangalore - Prof. of Medical Demography, Centre for Population Studies London School of Hygiene and Tropical Medicine, London, U.K.
86. Background paper to review current socio-economic factors affecting maternal mortality - Social Development Department - Overseas Development Administration UK., Zoe Oxaal & Veroniq Filippi.
87. Immediate and proximate causes of Maternal Mortality (Samce Maine 1992/Royston89).

88. An analytical model of Maternal Mortality (Maine and McCarthy - Tinker and Koblinsky)1993.

89. Statistical problems associated with the measurement of maternal mortality.

90. Relationship between socio-demographic factors and child survival : Evidences from Goa - India. T.S. Syamala, Institute for Social and Economic Change - Nagarbhavl Bangalore.

91. Demographic study of Gujjars of Delhi-VI factors affecting fertility, Infant Mortality and use of BCM, Sweta Dabral and S.L. Malik - Department of Anthropology (University of Delhi - Delhi-7, India).

92. Development is not essential to reduce infant mortality rate in India - experience from the Ballabgarh Project, J. Epidemiol, Community Health 2000, 247-253.

93. Millennium Development Goals - 4 & 5 indicators (MDG). (Improving Maternal, New Born & Child Health in the South East Asia Region.

94. Harvard Centre for Population and Development Studies, neonatal mortality in India - emerging Paradoxes - K.S. James - Ian Aitken, S.V. Subramanian (HCPDS - Working Paper Series Vol. 10 Number 13) November 2000, K.S. James - Centre for Eco. & Soc. Studies Nizamiah Observatory Campus, Begumpet, Hyderabad-500016.

95. The Australian National University Demography Program - Research School of Social Sciences. Determinants of Infant Mortality in a Backward Region of North India - Are Socio-economic or Demography factors Dominant? Santosh Jatrana (Working papers in Demography No. 82-1999).

96. Infant mortality in a Backward region of North India. Does Ethnicity matter? Santosh Jatrana, Asian Meta Centre for Population and Sustainable Development Analysis, Hd. Qrts. at Asia Research Institute - National University of Singapore.

97. Reducing Child Mortality in India in the New Millennium : Mariam Claeson, Eduard R. Bos, Tazim Mawji, and Indra Pathmanathan (World Bank Washington D.C. USA).

98. Ministry of Health and Family Welfare, Government of India - Annual Report 2005-2006.

99. Compendium of Research Projects in RCH (Min. of Health Family Welfare, Government of India).

100. National Rural Health Mission - Mission Document Mininstry of Health & Family Welfare - Government of India.

101. Janani Suraksha Yojana.

102. National Family Health Survey (1992-1993)

   (i) Maharashtra (MCH & Family Planning, Gokhale Instt. of PH. & Eco. Pune and International Instt. of Pop-sciences - Bombay November 1994.

   (ii) Haryana - NFHS. (1993).

   (iii) Rajasthan -1998-99. International Institute of Population Sciences - Mumbai.

   (iv) Andhra Pradesh

   (v) Tamil Nadu

103. 11th Five year Plan approach Paper : Infant Mortality Rate in 1990 (2003) Recent years. Best State : 11 per 1000 livebirths. Worst State in recent years : 83, maternal mortality (Per 1000 livebirths).

104. Search for a Vision Statement on Women's Empowerment vis-a-vis Legislation and Judicial Decisions. Sponsored by the National Commission for Women (Prepared by the Indian Trust for Innovation and Social Change, (ed: Padma Seth, 2004).

INDEX